Dysphagia in Adults and Children

Editors

MAUSUMI NATALIE SYAMAL
EILEEN M. RAYNOR

OTOLARYNGOLOGIC CLINICS OF NORTH AMERICA

www.oto.theclinics.com

Consulting Editor
SUJANA S. CHANDRASEKHAR

August 2024 • Volume 57 • Number 4

ELSEVIER

1600 John F. Kennedy Boulevard • Suite 1800 • Philadelphia, Pennsylvania, 19103-2899

http://www.oto.theclinics.com

OTOLARYNGOLOGIC CLINICS OF NORTH AMERICA Volume 57, Number 4
August 2024 ISSN 0030-6665, ISBN-13: 978-0-443-29644-4

Editor: Stacy Eastman
Developmental Editor: Malvika Shah

Otolaryngologic Clinics of North America (ISSN 0030-6665) is published bimonthly by Elsevier, Inc., 360 Park Avenue South, New York, NY 10010-1710. Months of issue are February, April, June, August, October, and December. Business and Editorial Offices: 1600 John F. Kennedy Blvd., Suite 1800, Philadelphia, PA 19103-2899. Customer Service Office: 6277 Sea Harbor Drive, Orlando, FL 32887-4800. Periodicals postage paid at New York, NY and additional mailing offices. Subscription prices are $478.00 per year (US individuals), $100.00 per year (US & Canadian student/resident), $623.00 per year (Canadian individuals), $679.00 per year (international individuals), $270.00 per year (international student/resident). For institutional access pricing please contact Customer Service via the contact information below. Foreign air speed delivery is included in all *Clinics'* subscription prices. All prices are subject to change without notice. **POSTMASTER:** Send address changes to *Otolaryngologic Clinics of North America*, Elsevier Health Sciences Division, Subscription Customer Service, 3251 Riverport Lane, Maryland Heights, MO 63043. **Telephone: 1-800-654-2452 (U.S. and Canada); 314-447-8871 (outside U.S. and Canada). Fax: 314-447-8029. E-mail: journalscustomerservice-usa@elsevier.com (for print support); journalsonlinesupport-usa@elsevier.com (for online support).**

Reprints. For copies of 100 or more of articles in this publication, please contact the Commercial Reprints Department, Elsevier Inc., 360 Park Avenue South, New York, NY 10010-1710. Tel.: 212-633-3874; Fax: 212-633-3820; E-mail: reprints@elsevier.com.

Otolaryngologic Clinics of North America is also published in Spanish by McGraw-Hill Interamericana Editores S.A., P.O. Box 5-237, 06500 Mexico D.F., Mexico.

Otolaryngologic Clinics of North America is covered in *MEDLINE/PubMed (Index Medicus), Current Contents/Clinical Medicine, Excerpta Medica, BIOSIS, Science Citation Index,* and *ISI/BIOMED.*

Contributors

CONSULTING EDITOR

SUJANA S. CHANDRASEKHAR, MD, FAAO-HNS, FAOS, FACS
Consulting Editor, Otolaryngologic Clinics of North America, President, American
Otological Society, Past President, American Academy of Otolaryngology–Head
and Neck Surgery, Partner, ENT & Allergy Associates, LLP, Clinical Professor,
Department of Otolaryngology–Head and Neck Surgery, Zucker School of Medicine at
Hofstra–Northwell, Hempstead, New York; Clinical Associate Professor, Department of
Otolaryngology–Head and Neck Surgery, Icahn School of Medicine at Mount Sinai,
New York, New York

EDITORS

MAUSUMI NATALIE SYAMAL, MD, MSE, FACS
Section Head, Laryngology, Director of the Rush Voice, Airway and Swallowing Program,
Assistant Professor, Department of Otorhinolaryngology, Division of Laryngology, Rush
University Medical Center, Chicago, Illinois

EILEEN M. RAYNOR, MD, FACS, FAAP
Chief, Division of Pediatric Otolaryngology, Associate Professor, HNSCS and Pediatrics,
Duke Department of Head and Neck Surgery and Communication Sciences, Duke Health
System, Duke University, Durham, North Carolina

AUTHORS

MELISSA ALLIBONE, MS, CCC-SLP
Speech Language Pathologist, Departments of Otorhinolaryngology–Head and Neck
Surgery, and Speech-Language Pathology, University of Pennsylvania, Philadelphia,
Pennsylvania

CRISTINA BALDASSARI, MD, FAAP, FACS
Professor, Department of Otolaryngology–Head and Neck Surgery, Eastern Virginia
Medical School, Department of Pediatric Sleep Medicine, Children's Hospital of the King's
Daughters, Norfolk, Virginia

MICHAEL BENNINGER, MD, FACS
Professor, Head and Neck Institute, Cleveland Clinic, Cleveland, Ohio; Cleveland Clinic
Voice Center

MARTIN B. BRODSKY, PhD, MSc, CCC-SLP
Head and Neck Institute, Cleveland Clinic, Cleveland, Ohio; Cleveland Clinic Voice Center;
Associate Professor, Department of Physical Medicine and Rehabilitation, Division of
Pulmonary and Critical Care Medicine, Johns Hopkins University, Baltimore, Maryland

PAUL C. BRYSON, MD, MBA, FACS
Associate Professor, Head and Neck Institute, Cleveland Clinic, Cleveland Clinic Voice Center, Cleveland, Ohio

SWAPNA K. CHANDRAN, MD
Professor, Department of Otolaryngology, Head and Neck Surgery and Communicative Disorders, University of Louisville, Louisville, Kentucky

ELLIANA KIRSH DEVORE, MD
Resident, Department of Otolaryngology–Head and Neck Surgery, Harvard Medical School, Division of Laryngology, Massachusetts Eye and Ear, Boston, Massachusetts

KARUNA DEWAN, MD, FACS
Associate Professor, Department of Otolaryngology–Head and Neck Surgery, Louisiana State University Health – Shreveport, Shreveport, Louisiana

MANON DOUCET, MD
Resident, Department of Otolaryngology, Head and Neck Surgery and Communicative Disorders, University of Louisville, Louisville, Kentucky

AMELIA F. DRAKE, MD
Distinguished Professor, Department of Otolaryngology–Head and Neck Surgery, University of North Carolina, Chapel Hill, North Carolina

ROSE P. EAPEN, MD
Chair of Otolaryngology, Long Beach Memorial, Pediatric Otolaryngology, Miller Children's Hospital, Manhattan Beach, California

ANNA ERMARTH, MD, MS
Assistant Professor, Department of Pediatrics, Division of Pediatric Gastroenterology, Hepatology and Nutrition, University of Utah School of Medicine, Salt Lake City, Utah

LAURENCE GASCON, MD, MSc, FRCSC
Head and Neck Institute, Cleveland Clinic, Fellow, Cleveland Clinic Voice Center, Cleveland, Ohio

ERIN R.S. HAMERSLEY, DO, CDR, MC, USN
Assistant Professor, Department of Otolaryngology–Head and Neck Surgery, Naval Medical Center, Portsmouth, Virginia; Department of Otolaryngology–Head and Neck Surgery, Eastern Virginia Medical School, Norfolk, Virginia

COURTNEY J. HUNTER, MD
Resident Physician, Department of Otolaryngology–Head and Neck Surgery, University of Arkansas for Medical Sciences, Little Rock, Arkansas

ALLISON KEANE, MD
Fellow, Department of Otolaryngology–Head and Neck Surgery, University of North Carolina, Chapel Hill, North Carolina

JENNIFER KERN, MS, CCC-SLP
Clinical Specialist in Speech Language Pathology, Duke Department of Speech Pathology and Audiology, Durham, North Carolina

DEEPAK LAKSHMIPATHY, BS
Clinical Research Fellow, Department of Otorhinolaryngology–Head and Neck Surgery, University of Pennsylvania, Philadelphia, Pennsylvania

ELTON LAMBERT, MD
Assistant Professor, Department of Otolaryngology, Baylor College of Medicine, Houston, Texas

JANET WAIMIN LEE, MD, FAAP
Assistant Professor, Department of Head and Neck Surgery and Communication Sciences, Division of Pediatric Otolaryngology, Duke University, Durham, North Carolina

LAUREN K. LEEPER, MD
Associate Professor, Department of Otolaryngology–Head and Neck Surgery, University of North Carolina, Chapel Hill, North Carolina

JORDYN LUCAS, MD
Assistant Professor, Department of Otolaryngology–Head and Neck Surgery, Eastern Virginia Medical School, Children's Hospital of the King's Daughters, Norfolk, Virginia

JORDAN LUTTRELL, MD
Resident, Department of Otolaryngology, University of Tennessee Health Science Center, Memphis, Tennessee

CHLOE SANTA MARIA, MD, MPH
Caruso Department of Otolaryngology Head and Neck Surgery, Clinical Instructor Physician, USC Voice Center, University of Southern California, Los Angeles, California

WADE MCCLAIN, DO
Assistant Professor, Department of Otolaryngology–Head and Neck Surgery, University of North Carolina, Chapel Hill, North Carolina

KARLA O'DELL, MD
Associate Professor, Caruso Department of Otolaryngology–Head and Neck Surgery, Assistant Professor, USC Voice Center, University of Southern California, Los Angeles, California

KRISTINA POWERS, MD
Resident Physician, Department of Otolaryngology–Head and Neck Surgery, Eastern Virginia Medical School, Norfolk, Virginia

KARTHIK RAJASEKARAN, MD, FACS
Assistant Professor, Department of Otorhinolaryngology–Head and Neck Surgery, Leonard Davis Institute of Health Economics, University of Pennsylvania, Philadelphia, Pennsylvania

EILEEN M. RAYNOR, MD, FACS, FAAP
Chief, Division of Pediatric Otolaryngology, Associate Professor, HNSCS and Pediatrics, Duke Department of Head and Neck Surgery and Communication Sciences, Duke Health System, Duke University, Durham, North Carolina

MILLER RICHMOND, MPH, MD
Resident Physician, Georgetown University School of Medicine, Washington, DC

MARISA A. RYAN, MD, MPH
Physician, Surgeon, Pediatric Otolaryngology, Peak ENT Associates, Provo, Utah

PHILLIP C. SONG, MD
Assistant Professor, Department of Otolaryngology–Head and Neck Surgery, Harvard Medical School, Director, Division of Laryngology, Massachusetts Eye and Ear, Boston, Massachusetts

JILLIAN NYSWONGER SUGG, MS, CCC-SLP
Speech Language Pathologist, Department of Head and Neck Surgery and Communication Sciences, Division of Speech Pathology and Audiology, Duke University, Durham, North Carolina

MAUSUMI NATALIE SYAMAL, MD, MSE, FACS
Section Head, Laryngology, Director of the Rush Voice, Airway and Swallowing Program, Assistant Professor, Department of Otorhinolaryngology, Division of Laryngology, Rush University Medical Center, Chicago, Illinois

MELIN TAN-GELLER, MD
Clinical Associate Professor, Department of Otorhinolaryngology–Head and Neck Surgery, Albert Einstein College of Medicine, Montefiore Medical Center, Bronx, New York

OZLEM E. TULUNAY-UGUR, MD
Patricia and J. Floyd Kyser, MD Professor in Otolaryngology Head and Neck Surgery, Director, Division of Laryngology, University of Arkansas for Medical Sciences, Little Rock, Arkansas

DANIEL WOHL, MD
Pediatric Otolaryngology Associates, Jacksonville, Florida

Contents

 Video content accompanies this article at http://www.oto.theclinics. com.

Swallowing problems in children can occur for a variety of reasons, and assessment varies based on the age of the child, underlying medical problems, and results of the clinical swallow evaluation. The need for interdisciplinary management with speech language pathologists skilled in the management of children with dysphagia is imperative to identify the components of swallowing that are impaired and provide specific recommendations for safe and adequate nutrition supporting growth, development, and oral feeding if possible. This study focuses on the types of assessment tools available and how and when they are utilized for children of different ages and abilities.

This article explores the landscape of dysphagia assessment in adults. Dysphagia, a complex condition affecting the lifespan and many health conditions, significantly compromises individuals' quality of life. Dysphagia is often underdiagnosed, emphasizing the need for comprehensive assessment methods to ensure timely and accurate intervention. It encompasses clinical history, physical examination, clinical and instrumental swallow evaluations. Procedures within each of these modalities are reviewed, highlighting strengths, limitations, and contribution toward a complete understanding of dysphagia, ultimately guiding effective intervention strategies for improved patient outcomes.

Pediatric dysphagia is a common condition encountered in clinical practice. We review the physiology and development of swallow, presentation, epidemiology, and etiology of dysphagia. Additionally, comorbidities, associated conditions, and medical management of dysphagia are discussed.

Patients with oral and pharyngeal dysphagia have difficulty forming a cohesive bolus and/or transferring food from the mouth into the pharynx and esophagus to initiate the involuntary swallowing process. This may be accompanied by nasopharyngeal regurgitation, aspiration, and a sensation of residual food remaining in the pharynx. Abnormalities affecting the upper esophageal sphincter, pharynx, larynx, or tongue, in isolation or combination, result in oropharyngeal dysphagia affecting either or both transit and airway protection. These issues can be addressed with a combination of management of the underlying systemic disease, with surgical intervention or with swallow therapy.

Oral causes of dysphagia in infancy may involve the lips, the tongue, or the palate. Whereas ankyloglossia is commonly diagnosed in infants with dysphagia, assessment of the need for surgical intervention may be less straightforward. Tongue size (macroglossia) may be associated with dysphagia as it may cause limitation of movement of the food or milk bolus by the lips or cheeks. Congenital conditions such as cleft lip and palate, micrognathia, or craniofacial microsomia may also be associated with dysphagia. Diagnosis and treatment of these conditions can be improved with the engagement of lactation and feeding experts as well as multidisciplinary craniofacial teams.

The upper aerodigestive system is closely intertwined from an embryologic and functional perspective. Laryngotracheal anatomic abnormalities, such as laryngomalacia, stenosis, vocal cord paralysis, and laryngeal clefts, affect not only the respiratory function but also the swallow function. Laryngotracheal pathology can interfere with the suck–swallow–breathe mechanism in infants. It can also exacerbate gastroesophageal reflux. Chronic aspiration secondary to laryngotracheal anomalies can result in respiratory and pulmonary complications. Surgical treatment of laryngotracheal anomalies can also cause transient or long-term swallow dysfunction. Multidisciplinary approaches and clinical assessment of swallowing are important in patients with laryngotracheal pathology.

Esophageal dysphagia is a common yet difficult to diagnose condition. This article underscores the role of detailed patient history and physical examinations, including prompt endoscopic evaluation, for accurate differentiation between esophageal and oropharyngeal dysphagia. The authors discuss the heightened importance of early intervention in certain patient groups, such as elderly individuals and patients with head and neck cancer, to mitigate the risk of malnutrition and infection. The authors delve into etiologic factors highlighting the complexity of clinical presentations and the significance of tailored management strategies.

Erin R.S. Hamersley and Cristina Baldassari

Swallowing is an elaborate process that requires neuromuscular coordination. Pediatric esophageal dysphagia is broadly categorized into structural and nonstructural causes. The structural causes of pediatric esophageal dysphagia are related to processes that narrow the lumen of the esophagus. Esophageal strictures are the result of scar tissue formation within the lumen of the esophagus, leading to stenosis. Vascular rings and slings cause external compression of the esophagus. Diagnosis requires an esophagram and computed tomography or magnetic resonance imaging. Treatment is guided by the patient's symptoms and underlying diagnosis, although it often requires surgical intervention when symptomatic.

Swapna K. Chandran and Manon Doucet

This article provides an overview of neurogenic dysphagia, describing the evaluation and management of swallowing dysfunction in various neurologic diseases. The article will focus on stroke, Parkinson's disease, amyotrophic lateral sclerosis, and multiple sclerosis.

Jillian Nyswonger Sugg and Janet Waimin Lee

Dysphagia is commonly associated with neurologic/neuromuscular disorders including prematurity, cerebral palsy, traumatic brain injury, brain tumors, genetic disorders, and neuromuscular diseases. This article aims to review the major categories of neurologic dysphagia, to outline specific findings and special considerations for each population, and to acknowledge the importance of integrating each patient's medical prognosis, goals of care, and developmental stage into a multidisciplinary treatment plan.

Mausumi Natalie Syamal

This manuscript reviews and outlines the necessary tools to efficiently assess and manage an adult patient where an esophageal foreign body is suspected. It reviews the vulnerable populations and relevant diagnostics and provides a triage diagram to aid in timely intervention. Management with esophagoscopy is reviewed as well as potential complications that may arise. Lastly, to illustrate the concepts of this section, a case study is presented to highlight the salient points.

Kristina Powers, Cristina Baldassari, and Jordyn Lucas

Foreign body ingestions commonly occur in children aged under 6 years. While serious complications of ingestions are rare, sharp objects, caustics, multiple magnets, and button batteries can be associated with poorer outcomes including gastrointestinal (GI) obstruction, perforation, necrosis, and fistula formation. Initial workup should include history, physical examination, and plain film radiographs that will identify radiopaque objects. Removal of the foreign body is typically warranted if the object is high risk, it is located higher up in the GI tract, the patient is symptomatic, or the object is retained for a prolonged amount of time.

Dysphagia is a common symptom in patients with head and neck cancer that can significantly impact health outcomes and quality of life. The origin of dysphagia in these patients is often multifactorial, making diagnosis and management especially complex. The evaluating otolaryngologist should be well versed with the patient's neoplasm, comorbidities, and treatment history alongside dysphagia-specific imaging modalities. Management is often dynamic, requiring frequent monitoring, interprofessional collaboration, and a variety of supportive and invasive measures to achieve optimal outcomes.

Children with tracheostomies have multiple challenges with respect to achieving normal deglutition. These children may have underlying neurologic or genetic conditions that can predispose to dysphagia, but even in children without underlying comorbidities, the presence of a tracheostomy tube impacts the mechanics of swallowing, leading to difficulty with different consistencies as well as management of normal oral secretions. Intubation prior to tracheostomy also impacts sensation in the upper aerodigestive tract increasing the risk of aspiration. Occlusion of the tracheostomy with a speaking valve or cap improves outcomes in swallow and prognosis for oral feeding.

Dysphagia is a common manifestation of endocrine and metabolic diseases. Swallowing is a complex neuromuscular process, with an interplay of sensory and motor function, that has voluntary and involuntary control. Disruptions in any of these processes can cause significant dysphagia. Endocrine disorders and metabolic derangements are systemic conditions that affect multiple organ systems. They contribute to the development of neuropathies, myopathies, and motility disorders that lead to swallowing difficulty. Malnutrition and critical illness can lead to deconditioning and atrophy which can cause dysphagia, which in turn can lead to further malnutrition and deconditioning.

Gastroesophageal reflux (GER) and eosinophilic esophagitis (EoE) are the most common inflammatory causes of pediatric dysphagia, but several other less prevalent conditions should be considered. These conditions can affect one or several aspects of the swallowing process. In some inflammatory conditions dysphagia may be an early symptom. Esophagoscopy and instrumental swallow studies are often needed to determine the underlying diagnosis and best treatment plan. In some inflammatory conditions dysphagia can portend a worse outcome and need for more aggressive treatment of the underlying condition. Consultations with speech language pathology, gastroenterology, dietetics, allergy/immunology and/or rheumatology are often needed to optimize management.

Older adults are projected to outnumber children aged under 18 years for the first time in United States history by 2034, according to Census Bureau projections. This will lead to significant increase in age-related disorders. One of the most important disorders that will increase in prevalence is dysphagia, as it leads to malnutrition, dehydration, aspiration pneumonia, and death. In this article, the physiology of dysphagia in the elderly, as well as the management options is discussed.

While many patients who present with dysphagia have a clinically identifiable cause of dysphagia, the etiology of swallowing difficulty is oftentimes a diagnostic enigma. The aim of this article is to review possible etiologies of dysphagia when objective evidence of dysphagia is lacking. Included in this discussion are cricopharyngeal spasm, retrograde cricopharyngeal dysfunction, muscle tension dysphagia, dysphagia secondary to medications, and functional dysphagia.

OTOLARYNGOLOGIC CLINICS OF NORTH AMERICA

SERIES OF RELATED INTEREST

Facial Plastic Surgery Clinics
Available at: https://www.facialplastic.theclinics.com/

THE CLINICS ARE AVAILABLE ONLINE!
Access your subscription at:
www.theclinics.com

Foreword

Coordinating the Swallow in Children and Adults

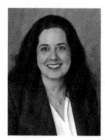

Sujana S. Chandrasekhar, MD, FACS, FAAO-HNS, FAOS
Consulting Editor

Swallowing seems so simple, but in reality, it is quite complex. As Drs Syamal and Raynor describe in their preface to this issue of *Otolaryngologic Clinics of North America*, the muscular and mucosal actions needed for a proper swallow are beautifully orchestrated like a ballet corps dancing to a symphony. The same elegant orchestration is needed between the health care providers identifying and managing the symptom. The *International Classification of Diseases, Tenth Revision (ICD-10)* coding system[1] classifies six separate codes for dysphagia: R13.10, R13.11, R13.12, R13.13, R13.14, and R13.19, relating to dysphagia, which is unspecified, oral phase, oropharyngeal phase, pharyngeal phase, pharyngoesophageal phase, and other, respectively. Issues relating to swallow are different in children and adults, as you will learn in this issue, and I commend the Guest Editors on assembling an outstanding set of articles and authors to cover the subject in detail.

Rather than separating this issue between children and adults, Drs Syamal and Raynor have interleaved the articles on each subject addressing the age groups. For example, assessing dysphagia poses different challenges depending on the age and cooperation capacity of the patient. Those articles following each other paint a more complete picture of the spectrum of possible causes. Similarly treated are the subsites of dysphagia, as well as neurologic dysphagia. We often limit our thinking of foreign body and caustic ingestion to children, but adults face this issue as well. The issue continues on to address swallowing issues related to other diagnoses, including head and neck cancer and its treatments, children with tracheostomy, endocrine and metabolic issues, and inflammation. "Adults" are lumped between ages 18 and over 100 years of age, but we are all aware that medical issues affect individuals in the geriatric age group, both elderly and older elderly, differently. Ergo, the inclusion of an article

https://doi.org/10.1016/j.otc.2024.04.004

addressing this group. The issue concludes with an article on the most challenging scenarios. The complex of the complex, as it were.

I thought we took a bit of a chance combining assessment and management of dysphagia in all age groups in one issue, and I commend Drs Syamal and Raynor and all of the authors featured in this issue of *Otolaryngologic Clinics of North America*, on meeting and exceeding the challenge. I find this issue to be an excellent resource for all of the "dancers"—otolaryngologists, speech and swallow therapists (or pathologists), radiologists, gastroenterologists, neurologists, pediatricians, internists, and family physicians—to be able to help the patient coordinate this complex, beautiful, and often overlooked symphonic function.

Sujana S. Chandrasekhar, MD, FACS, FAAO-HNS, FAOS
Consulting Editor
Otolaryngologic Clinics of North America
President
American Otological Society
Past President
American Academy of Otolaryngology–
Head and Neck Surgery
Partner, ENT & Allergy Associates, LLP

Clinical Professor
Department of Otolaryngology–
Head and Neck Surgery
Zucker School of Medicine at Hofstra–Northwell

Clinical Associate Professor
Department of Otolaryngology–
Head and Neck Surgery
Icahn School of Medicine at Mount Sinai
18 East 48th Street, 2nd Floor
New York, NY 10017, USA

E-mail address:
ssc@nyotology.com

REFERENCE

1. Centers for Medicare and Medicaid Services: billing and coding: swallowing studies for dysphagia. Available at: https://www.cms.gov/medicare-coverage-database/view/article.aspx?articleid=56621&ver=19&. [Accessed 6 April 2024].

Preface

Dysphagia: A Symphony of Senses at the Ballet Takes a Turn...

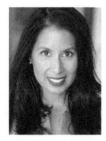 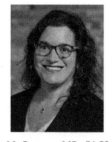

Mausumi Natalie Syamal, MD, MSE, FACS   Eileen M. Raynor, MD, FACS, FAAP
Editors

Ah Dysphagia! I have a love-hate relationship with dysphagia. I will start with what I love: the act of deglutition. I love it like Stanley Tucci loves travelling through Italy showing us the recipe of the first Bolognese by Artusi. I love that it involves nearly all our senses. The sight, the aroma, the textures, and tastes are like a symphony! I love that it even invokes a sixth sense of proprioception, as Anthony Bourdain felt that food tasted better barefoot on the sand. I often describe to my patients that swallowing is like a complex choreographed ballet. When performed properly, it is effortless and artful. However, when it goes awry, which for most of us it will at some point, I hate it. The usual joy and rituals of eating and sharing meals become cumbersome. Social connections wane along with nutritional status. All the senses suffer. The joy of eating becomes more of a chore. Like the injured ballet dancer who struggles on pointe and becomes dizzy, the dance is no longer effortless. The symphony seems cacophonous, even though the memory of flawless deglutition remains and that becomes painful to bear. Mostly, I hate that we cannot always cure dysphagia but only help manage it for some patients.

In this issue of *Otolaryngologic Clinics of North America*, we review dysphagia in both the adult and the child by underlying etiology. Each section serves as a guide to help the Otolaryngologist consider the many tools available for workup and management. Some excellent decision tree diagrams for differential diagnoses, assessment, and foreign body management are provided. Dysphagia assessment questionnaires specific to neurologic etiologies are mentioned. Newer treatment options and considerations, such as the effect of GLP-1 agonist drugs and Functional Lumen Imaging Probe and Peroral Endoscopic Myotomy, are discussed as well. We investigate special conditions that impact deglutition, such as children with a tracheostomy or with neurodevelopmental and craniofacial challenges. I will admit that in the process of editing

Otolaryngol Clin N Am 57 (2024) xv–xvi
https://doi.org/10.1016/j.otc.2024.02.022
oto.theclinics.com

this issue, I walked away feeling better about dysphagia. It is my hope that whether you love or hate dysphagia, this issue will leave you knowing how to better help the dancer and restore some of the joyous symphony.

DISCLOSURES

M.N. Syamal has no commercial or financial conflicts of interest. E.M. Raynor has no conflicts of interest.

Mausumi Natalie Syamal, MD, MSE, FACS
Department of Otorhinolaryngology
Rush University Medical Center
1611 West Harrison Street, Suite 550
Chicago, IL 60612, USA

Eileen M. Raynor, MD, FACS, FAAP
Division of Pediatric Otolaryngology
Department of Head and Neck Surgery &
Communication Sciences
Duke University
DUMC Box 3805
Durham, NC 27710, USA

E-mail addresses:
Mausumi_N_Syamal@rush.edu (M.N. Syamal)
Eileen.raynor@duke.edu (E.M. Raynor)

Assessing Dysphagia in the Child

Eileen M. Raynor, MD[a],*, Jennifer Kern, MS, CCC-SLP[b,1]

KEYWORDS

- Swallow • Dysphagia • Breast-feeding • Bottle-feeding • Video swallow • VFSS
- FEES • Modified barium swallow

KEY POINTS

- Assessment of dysphagia varies based on age and clinical variables specific to each child.
- A clinical swallow evaluation can help determine if an instrumental swallow study is warranted and which study is most appropriate for the situation as well as the best timing for the study.
- Certain pediatric populations are at elevated risk for dysphagia and need to be evaluated early on by specialized feeding therapists.
- Feeding issues unrelated to dysphagia are prevalent in children and may require alternative methods for assessment and management.

 Video content accompanies this article at http://www.oto.theclinics.com.

INTRODUCTION

Feeding and swallowing in children is a dynamic, complex process impacted by anatomic, physiologic, and neurologic development. A disruption in any of these realms can lead to a feeding or swallowing problem. Prior to 2019, there was not a universally agreed upon term to label feeding difficulties which is necessary to advance clinical practice, research, and policy; however, in 2019, a consensus definition and conceptual framework was proposed for "pediatric feeding disorder."[1,2] A pediatric feeding disorder has been defined as "impaired oral intake that is not age appropriate, and is associated with medical, nutritional, feeding skills, and/or psychosocial dysfunction."[1] Given the multiple underlying mechanisms that can contribute to pediatric feeding disorders, interdisciplinary care is critical for an effective assessment and treatment.[2,3] The focus of this study is on the assessment of pediatric dysphagia and

[a] Duke Department of Head and Neck Surgery & Communication Sciences, DUMC Box 3805, Durham, NC 27710, USA; [b] Duke Department of Speech Pathology & Audiology, DUMC Box 3887, Durham, NC 27710, USA
[1] Present address: 12204 Queensbridge Court, Raleigh, NC 27613.
* Corresponding author. 2212 Timberview Drive, Durham, NC 27705.
E-mail address: Eileen.raynor@duke.edu

Otolaryngol Clin N Am 57 (2024) 511–521
https://doi.org/10.1016/j.otc.2024.02.011

will therefore focus on the assessment of the skills component of a pediatric feeding disorder.

Critical components of a pediatric clinical swallow evaluation remain consistent across ages; however, the specific swallowing components that are evaluated vary based on the age and skill level of the child given the changes that occur over time with anatomy, physiology, and diet expectations. Infants are obligate nasal breathers and require the coordination of the "suck, swallow, and breathe" cycles for successful oral feeding. Difficulties with the coordination of sucking, swallowing, and breathing can affect a child's overall health, growth, and development. Other variables unique to early infancy are that all of the phases of the swallow are reflexive in nature,[3] and diet consists of a single consistency, liquid. Infants may be exclusively breast-fed, exclusively bottle-fed, or both breast-fed and bottle-fed, therefore it is important to assess feeding and swallowing abilities across modalities as there may be significant differences.[4–6] Later in infancy, the oral phase of the swallow becomes voluntary, which is critical for the advancement of oral motor skills for safe manipulation of solids.[3] As children advance in gross motor development, spoon-feeding and cup drinking are introduced until ultimately a diet consists of a variety of solid food textures via various utensils. Safe swallowing requires the integration of timely sensory information and coordinated motor responses. A variety of conditions such as neurodevelopmental diagnoses, anatomic abnormalities, genetic conditions, and other comorbidities affecting the aerodigestive tract can impact feeding and swallowing abilities and contribute to problems such as aspiration or poor growth.[7,8]

DEFINITIONS

Phases of swallowing: It is difficult to clearly distinguish the starting and endings points of the specific phases of swallowing given the dynamic nature of the swallowing mechanism. Below is a description of the various phases of the swallow. Any one or several of these phases may be impacted contributing to a diagnosis of dysphagia.

Oral phase: Food or liquid is introduced into the mouth, formed into a cohesive bolus, and then propelled posteriorly in the oral cavity toward the pharynx. Conditions affecting the oral phase include cleft palate, micrognathia, ankyloglossia, oral motor weakness, macroglossia, and facial paralysis.[9–11]

Oropharyngeal phase: This is the phase where the swallow reflex is initiated. The elevation of the soft palate and the posterior movement of the base of tongue propel the bolus in anticipation of a swallow. The larynx elevates, the vocal cords adduct, and the epiglottis retroflexes to protect the airway from the incoming bolus. Conditions impacting the oropharyngeal phase include cleft palate, laryngomalacia, laryngeal cleft, vocal cord paralysis, micrognathia, retrognathia, and masses involving the base of tongue.[12–15]

Pharyngoesophageal phase: The pharyngeal constrictor muscles squeeze to push the bolus inferiorly to the upper esophageal sphincter that relaxes to allow entry into the esophagus. The larynx remains closed during this portion of the swallow. Low muscle tone, neurologic conditions, laryngeal cleft, tight upper esophageal sphincter, cricopharyngeal bar, and pharyngeal masses can all impact this phase of swallowing.[16,17]

Esophageal phase: The bolus is transported through the esophagus via peristalsis from the upper esophageal sphincter through the lower esophageal sphincter into the stomach. The larynx relaxes for respiration and the system is ready for the next oral bite or sip. Conditions that can impact esophageal motility include tracheoesophageal fistulae, esophageal stenosis, inflammatory conditions of the esophagus, retroesophageal innominate artery or vascular rings, and severe gastroesophageal reflux disease.[18–20]

Laryngeal penetration: The bolus enters the laryngeal vestibule to the level of the vocal folds but does not go below the vocal folds into the airway. The bolus is typically expelled into the pharynx.

Laryngeal aspiration: The bolus enters the laryngeal vestibule below the level of the vocal folds into the trachea. Aspiration may trigger a sensory response such as cough or throat clear or there may be the absence of a sensory response (silent aspiration).[5,12]

SIGNS AND SYMPTOMS OF DYSPHAGIA

Neonates present with unique signs of dysphagia compared to older infants/children given the reflexive nature of sucking in early infancy. Signs of dysphagia in this population may include eye watering, facial grimace, breath holding, physiologic decompensation (bradycardia, desaturation), tachypnea, stridor, sleep feeding, audible congestion, anterior spill, and coughing/choking during oral feeding. Of note, in infants and young children with dysphagia and aspiration, silent aspiration is more common than that of aspiration with a sensory response.[5,7,21] This can be attributed to the laryngeal chemoreflex not yet having reached maturity which is a primary defensive mechanism for prevention and/or protection (cough response) from airway invasion.[6,7,15] As sucking reflexes are integrated, refusal behaviors such as turning/pulling away from bottle/breast may emerge as signs of dysphagia. Other signs include prolonged mealtimes, congestion, eye watering, coughing, choking, gagging, and emesis. As children begin transitioning to purees and solid foods, symptoms may include anterior loss, expelling food, gagging, food refusal, refusals of specific textures, prolonged mastication, prolonged mealtimes, pocketing, or coughing and choking. Children with heightened oral sensation may have difficulties tolerating specific textures and may limit their diet to those textures they feel the safest with. Older children who can describe symptoms with verbal language may describe the feeling of something "being stuck."

EVALUATION

Evaluation of pediatric dysphagia is completed by a speech language pathologist (SLP) with specialized training in feeding and swallowing and is individualized based on the age, diet, and underlying condition of the patient presenting.

Clinical swallow evaluation: This evaluation is typically completed as a first step in the assessment process to gather information regarding the child's feeding and swallowing abilities and to establish a functional baseline and determine whether and when further instrumental assessment or other referrals are warranted. A clinical swallow evaluation begins with a thorough history and includes an oral mechanical evaluation, observation of a typical feeding or meal including caregiver–child interaction, motor patterns, and behaviors surrounding mealtime. During the evaluation, the clinician will implement intervention strategies to determine the impact on feeding and swallowing to provide additional information regarding swallowing dysfunction and the response to the strategy trialed (ie, utensils, positioning, external pacing, and cue-based feeding).[3,5,21] A primary benefit of the clinical swallow evaluation is that it includes an observation of a typical feeding from beginning to completion in a context similar to that of the home environment compared to instrumental studies. This often results in greater participation and can result in better data collection than with instrumental assessments requiring alteration of food/liquid presented and or use of endoscope. Clinical signs of aspiration may be subtle such as eye watering, arching, observable delay in swallow initiation, or stridor or overt such as coughing and choking. Poor growth or respiratory illness may be symptoms of dysphagia.[2–4]

Common Instrumental Swallowing Evaluations

1. Video fluoroscopic swallow study (VFSS): The goal of the VFSS is to evaluate swallow function, swallowing efficiency, and airway protection. A VFSS should only be completed on infants and children with a suspect or confirmed swallowing dysfunction, the ability and readiness to participate, and when findings will impact the treatment plan.[22–24] This study is performed in a radiology suite where a variety of consistencies are mixed with barium and presented to the child. The infant or child is typically positioned on the fluoroscopy table (elevated side-lying positioning) or upright in a supportive seating device/chair and x-ray fluoroscopy is utilized in real time to evaluate the swallow in the lateral and/or anterior and posterior (AP) positions. One benefit of the VFSS is that it allows for direct observation of all phases of the swallow from oral through esophageal phases.[25,26] VFSS can identify whether anatomic abnormalities are present, provide information regarding various components of swallowing function including motor movement, timing, coordination, and sensation. Some examples of swallowing components assessed in this study include velar elevation, tongue base retraction, opening of upper esophageal sphincter, presence of airway invasion, and presence or absence and efficacy of a sensory response, as well as the response to various interventions trialed during the study (Video 1 and 2).

2. Fiberoptic endoscopic evaluation of swallow (FEES): This study is performed using a flexible endoscope passed transnasally allowing for visualization of the nasopharynx and hypopharynx while the infant or child is actively swallowing. Food coloring is sometimes used to provide better identification of the liquid or solid bolus and distinguish from bodily secretions. This study allows for visualization leading up to and immediately following the swallow with a white out period during the swallow due to epiglottic inversion.[2,22] FEES provides information regarding anatomic differences, asymmetry of movement, location of bolus at time of swallow initiation (ie, vallecula, pyriform sinus, and aryepiglottic folds) including the presence and efficacy of a sensory response to laryngeal penetration or aspiration. It also provides information regarding quantity and location of laryngeal residue post-swallow. Overt laryngopharyngeal reflux may also be observed with this modality. An additional benefit of FEES for nonoral or minimally oral feeders is the ability to gather information regarding swallowing of secretions.[27,28] In addition, there is no time restriction in a FEES study as there is with VFSS allowing for potential observation of the entirety of a meal to detect changes in swallow function with fatigue and with a variety of food consistencies (Video 3).

Deciding which assessment to pursue can be challenging as each has different benefits and limitations. Efforts to develop a screening tool that can assist clinicians as to the best options for the evaluation of dysphagia in children have been ongoing. There is a promising tool pediatric screening–priority evaluation dysphagia (PS-PED) that has demonstrated good concordance with VFSS evaluations and does not require feeding the child to administer. This in addition to a clinical swallow evaluation may allow for better decision-making as to the next steps in the dysphagia workup.[29] The flow chart shown in **Fig. 1** can serve as a tool to help with the decision-making process. In general, if the clinical swallowing evaluation indicates dysphagia isolated to the oral phrase or nondysphagia feeding difficulties, then feeding therapy or additional referrals are potentially indicated. For situations where there is concern about airway protection or pharyngeal dysphagia, instrumented studies are beneficial to direct the next steps of treatment.[2,22] A significant difference in clinical practice between adult and pediatric populations is the very important factor of patient participation in instrumental studies.

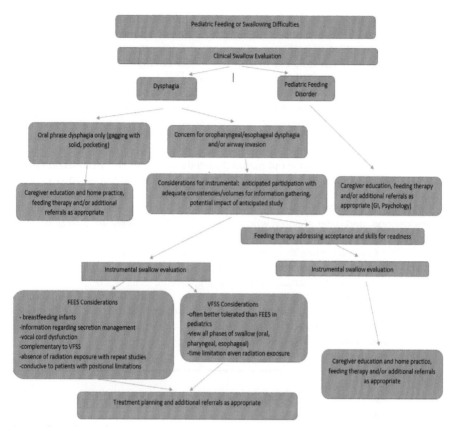

Fig. 1. Flow chart of assessment options in the setting of pediatric dysphagia.

It is a common occurrence where an instrumental study would be beneficial clinically, but the child is not accepting adequate volumes and/or likely to participate in the study therefore not making it a viable option.[30–32] In these instances, the clinician must rely on information from clinical assessment and communication with the medical team while addressing acceptance of various oral presentations in feeding therapy. Furthermore, given that a swallowing evaluation provides information regarding one point in time, that information must be placed in the context of the larger clinical picture when making treatment recommendations. **Fig. 1** is a flow chart to help guide clinical decision-making for the type of feeding and swallowing assessment most appropriate for a given patient.

CHALLENGES

Of course, each of the options for evaluating swallowing has limitations. Limitations of the clinical swallow evaluation include subjectivity related to clinician training and experience, reliance on the child's hunger and/or participation, and the prevalence of silent aspiration in the pediatric population. Despite the many benefits of the VFSS, it carries the risk of radiation exposure given the use of fluoroscopy. In an effort to limit radiation exposure, time under active fluoroscopy, frames/seconds captured, and clarity of the image may be inadequate to provide clear visualization of the laryngotracheal complex or the ability to capture aspiration events across the entirety of a feeding/meal. Other limitations include positioning of a patient and participation in acceptance/swallowing of barium. Furthermore, it is important to note that while the VFSS does provide information regarding bolus flow throughout the esophagus, it is not a complete assessment of esophageal function.[19,25] There are important initiatives underway to standardize infant and pediatrics VFSS protocols and documentation to decrease radiation exposure, improve information exchange among studies, and determine measurable intervention.[23,33,34] Some of the limitations of pediatric FEES include participation given the discomfort associated with the endoscope, movement of the head and body affecting clarity of the video imaging, nasal regurgitation impacting visualization of larynx, white out period during the swallow, and visualization of the pharyngeal phase of the swallow only. The groups of pediatric populations who are typically the most successful with FEES are young infants during the reflexive sucking period, children with altered sensation who are likely to remain still during passing of the endoscope, and older children who are likely to stay relatively still and participate in eating/drinking during the study with coaching and support from clinicians and caregivers.[28,30,31] Given the benefits and limitation of these assessment modalities, multiple studies can be complementary to one another and serve to provide the whole picture of the swallow mechanism. Technical and clinical skills of the SLP performing the study and in the case of the VFSS along with the technical skills of the radiologist are paramount to obtaining a reliable assessment. **Boxes 1** and **2** describe the swallowing components assessed during VFSS and a Penetration-Aspiration Scale frequently used in both VFSS and FEES.

Box 1
Swallowing components assessed during video fluoroscopic swallow study*

Lip closure or labial seal

Oral control of bolus

Mastication or bolus formation

Lingual bolus transport

Oral residue

Initial laryngeal elevation

Pharyngeal swallow initiation

Anterior hyoid motion

Peak laryngeal vestibular closure

Epiglottic movement

Soft palate elevation

Tongue base retraction

Pharyngeal stripping wave

Pharyngeal residue

Upper esophageal sphincter opening

Bolus flow through esophagus

*Of note, all components do not apply to all pediatric patients due to anatomic and physiologic differences across ages. There are also additional components not listed specific to bottle-feeding.

> **Box 2**
> **Penetration-aspiration scale**
>
> 1. Material does not enter airway.
> 2. Material enters airway, remains above the vocal folds, and is ejected from the airway.
> 3. Material enters the airway, remains above the vocal folds, and is not ejected from the airway.
> 4. Material enters the airway, contacts the vocal folds, and is ejected from the airway.
> 5. Material enters the airway, contacts the vocal folds, and is not ejected from the airway.
> 6. Material enters the airway, passes below the vocal folds, and is ejected into the larynx or out of the airway.
> 7. Material enters the airway, passes below the vocal folds, and is not ejected from the trachea despite effort.
> 8. Material enters the airway, passes below the vocal folds, and no effort is made to eject.
>
> *From* Rosenbek JC, Robbins JA, Roecker EB, Coyle JL, Wood JL. A penetration-aspiration scale. Dysphagia 1996;11:93-98.

Study Interpretation

Efforts have been made to standardize the interpretation and reporting of instrumented swallow studies by describing each of the components of swallowing using abnormalities that may influence the ultimate finding of either aspiration or laryngeal penetration.[33,34] Clear communication between the SLP performing the study within the report is critical to the treating speech pathologist and the ordering providers to determine best diet and intervention recommendations and additional referrals.

Other Feeding Considerations

Many children have feeding difficulties that are not associated with dysphagia. A pediatric feeding disorder is a unifying term for any feeding difficulty within the 4 areas of medical, nutritional, feeding skill, and psychosocial concerns.[1] This may include a child with oral hypersensitivity resulting in limited volumes or solid food textures, pocketing or expelling food, or gagging with foods. Feeding therapy via a variety of professionals (occupational therapist, SLP, and psychologist) is typically the best way to manage these issues. In extreme cases, children may require gastrostomy supplementation for nutrition.[2,6,29]

Special Conditions

1. *Cleft palate*: A cleft palate can impact the oral and pharyngeal phases of swallowing due to reduced compression and suction for extraction of liquids and the presence of nasal regurgitation. Children with a cleft palate often benefit from use of a specialty compression-based bottle system, specific positioning, and additional strategies to maximize comfort and efficiency. Of note, children with a cleft lip alone without palatal involvement generally feed well via breast-feeding or use of a standard bottle as they are able to generate adequate negative pressure with the tongue palate seal without the need for complete lip seal.[10] Micrognathia and other craniofacial syndromes that impact the palate and mandible can also create issues with feeding throughout childhood and may require several assessments and interventions over time.[11]

2. *Neurodevelopmental disorders*: A variety of conditions can impact motor and/or sensory functions across the phases of swallowing. Depending on the severity of the condition, these children may require supplemental gastrostomy feeds. Down syndrome, hypoxic ischemic encephalopathy, seizures disorders, muscular dystrophy, and traumatic brain injury are some of the more common conditions within this category. Consideration of instrumental swallowing evaluation is critical when appropriate in this population of patients as silent aspiration is common.[5,16,21,24,35] A study by Jackson found that 90.2% of children with Down syndrome who demonstrated aspiration on a VFSS, did so silently.[17]

3. *Vocal fold immobility*: Reduced vocal fold mobility may be due to cardiac procedures such as patent ductus arteriosis (PDA) ligation or aortic arch surgery, Chiari malformation, iatrogenic injury, or idiopathic. Children with vocal fold paralysis are at risk for aspiration due to incomplete closure of the glottis during swallow initiation. Positioning and potentially thickening of liquids may be necessary to assure adequate and safe nutrition intake orally.[13,21] Laryngomalacia is also a risk factor for aspiration due to floppy supraglottic structures interfering with normal laryngeal function during swallow. In a systematic review, dysphagia in these babies approached 50%.[14,36,37]

4. *Tracheostomy*: Children who are tracheostomy dependent may be at higher risk for dysphagia given the potential alterations to physiologic and biomechanical aspects of the swallow.[38,39] Use of a 1 way speaking valve or a cap if tolerated during swallowing can restore the subglottic pressure, reduce risk of aspiration, improve olfaction, and improve secretion management.[40,41]

5. *Oral restriction*: There is growing evidence to support that ankyloglossia can contribute to caregiver discomfort, aerophagia, and oral dysphagia in breast-feeding infants.[9,42] Ultrasound studies have demonstrated that breast-feeding relies primarily on the creation of intraoral negative pressure consisting of both tongue elevation and a sucking motion associated with movement of both the anterior and midtongue together to create that intraoral pressure.[43] Therefore, it is important to assess tongue elevation and movement of anterior and medial aspect of the tongue during sucking. A diagnosis of a tethered or tied tissue alone does not indicate a functional impact on feeding.[9] A comprehensive evaluation of feeding skills is necessary to determine functional impact of tethered oral tissues. There is conflicting evidence regarding the potential functional impact of tethered labial frenulae on infant feeding skills and gastrointestinal discomfort. Additionally, there is little-to-no correlation between tethered labial frenulae and breast-feeding success rates.[44] Assessment of lingual lateralization is also important when assessing for tethered oral tissues as a child is older and eating table foods as that movement is critical for mastication and clearance of residue from dentition and buccal cavities. Retrognathia and micrognathia are conditions that result in a superior and posterior lingual placement that can impact latch and efficiency with extraction and contribute to palatal crowding and development of a high arched palate which may also impact oral phase dysphagia.[10,11]

DISCUSSION

Assessment of swallowing in children requires a thorough understanding of the sensory and motor aspects of the phases of swallowing and the impact of any underlying conditions on swallow function. Identification of dysphagia, determination of the specific components of swallowing that are impacted, and understanding a child's overall medical, psychosocial, and nutritional variables can facilitate the most effective therapeutic interventions tailored to the individual. Both clinical and instrumental assessments of swallowing play important roles in gathering information to direct feeding and swallowing recommendations and treatment. No one assessment type is the preferred method for evaluation of all pediatric feeding disorders, and careful thought should be applied to which assessment type is the most appropriate at a given time for that specific child, based on presentation and information needed. There is more research to be done with standardization of assessment and report of results from pediatric instrumented swallowing assessments to support reliability and communication of information across studies and medical professionals. Given the complexity of medical, motor, sensory, nutritional, and social aspects that can impact eating, best clinical practice involves care from an interdisciplinary team of professionals.

Eating is one of life's greatest pleasures. And although not all children will be able to eat completely by mouth, the goal is for every child to have a safe and positive experience with mealtimes when at all possible.

CLINICS CARE POINTS

- Assessment of feeding and swallowing in children is different depending on the child's stage of development from infancy, toddler, childhood, and adolescence.
- Medical and genetic conditions may affect feeding and swallowing in a variety of ways.
- Specialized training in swallowing assessments and standardization of reporting results will improve care and therapeutic interventions.
- In pediatrics, participation is one of the primary factors impacting a clinician's ability to complete a comprehensive assessment of swallowing including instrumental swallow studies.

DISCLOSURE

The authors have nothing to disclose.

SUPPLEMENTARY DATA

Supplementary data to this article can be found online at https://doi.org/10.1016/j.otc. 2024.02.011.

REFERENCES

1. Goday PS, Huh SY, Silverman A, et al. Pediatric feeding disorder: consensus definition and conceptual framework. J Pediatr Gastroenterol Nutr 2019;68(1):124–9.
2. Arvedson JC. Assessment of pediatric dysphagia and feeding disorders: clinical and instrumental approaches. Dev Disabil Res Rev 2008;14(2):118–27 (In eng).
3. Dodrill P, Gosa MM. Pediatric dysphagia: physiology, assessment, and management. Ann Nutr Metabol 2015;66(Suppl. 5):24–31.
4. Calvo I, Conway A, Henriques F, et al. Diagnostic accuracy of the clinical feeding evaluation in detecting aspiration in children: a systematic review. Dev Med Child Neurol 2016;58(6):541–53.
5. DeMatteo C, Matovich D, Hjartarson A. Comparison of clinical and videofluoroscopic evaluation of children with feeding and swallowing difficulties. Dev Med Child Neurol 2005;47(3):149–57.
6. Kakodkar K, Schroeder JW. Pediatric dysphagia. Pediatric Clinics 2013;60(4): 969–77.

7. Lefton-Greif MA. Pediatric dysphagia. Physical Medicine and Rehabilitation Clinics 2008;19(4):837–51.
8. Kamity R, Kapavarapu PK, Chandel A. Feeding problems and long-term outcomes in preterm infants—a systematic approach to evaluation and management. Children 2021;8(12):1158.
9. Hill RR, Lee CS, Pados BF. The prevalence of ankyloglossia in children aged <1 year: a systematic review and meta-analysis. Pediatr Res 2021;90(2):259–66 (In eng).
10. Miller CK. Feeding issues and interventions in infants and children with clefts and craniofacial syndromes. Seminars in speech and language. © Thieme Medical Publishers; 2011. p. 115–26.
11. van de Lande LS, Caron CJ, Pluijmers BI, et al. Evaluation of swallow function in patients with craniofacial microsomia: a retrospective study. Dysphagia 2018;33: 234–42.
12. Bae SO, Lee GP, Seo HG, et al. Clinical characteristics associated with aspiration or penetration in children with swallowing problem. Annals of rehabilitation medicine 2014;38(6):734–41.
13. Irace AL, Dombrowski ND, Kawai K, et al. Aspiration in children with unilateral vocal fold paralysis. Laryngoscope 2019;129(3):569–73.
14. Jaffal H, Isaac A, Johannsen W, et al. The prevalence of swallowing dysfunction in children with laryngomalacia: a systematic review. Int J Pediatr Otorhinolaryngol 2020;139:110464.
15. Prasse JE, Kikano GE. An overview of pediatric dysphagia. Clinical pediatrics 2009;48(3):247–51.
16. Caruso AM, Bommarito D, Girgenti V, et al. Evaluation of Dysphagia and Inhalation Risk in Neurologically Impaired Children Using Esophageal High-Resolution Manometry with Swallowing Analysis. Children 2022;9(12):1987.
17. Jackson A, Maybee J, Moran MK, et al. Clinical characteristics of dysphagia in children with Down syndrome. Dysphagia 2016;31:663–71.
18. Cheung KM, Oliver MR, Cameron DJ, et al. Esophageal eosinophilia in children with dysphagia. J Pediatr Gastroenterol Nutr 2003;37(4):498–503.
19. Lanzoni G, Sembenini C, Gastaldo S, et al. Esophageal dysphagia in children: state of the art and proposal for a symptom-based diagnostic approach. Frontiers in Pediatrics 2022;10:885308.
20. Rayyan M, Allegaert K, Omari T, et al. Dysphagia in children with esophageal atresia: current diagnostic options. Eur J Pediatr Surg 2015;25(4):326–32.
21. Linden P, Kuhlemeier K, Patterson C. The probability of correctly predicting subglottic penetration from clinical observations. Dysphagia 1993;8:170–9.
22. Arvedson JC, Lefton-Greif MA. Instrumental assessment of pediatric dysphagia. Seminars in speech and language. Thieme Medical Publishers; 2017. p. 135–46.
23. Lefton-Greif MA, McGrattan KE, Carson KA, et al. First Steps Towards Development of an Instrument for the Reproducible Quantification of Oropharyngeal Swallow Physiology in Bottle-Fed Children. Dysphagia 2018;33(1):76–82 (In eng).
24. Chou Y, Wang L-W, Lin C-J, et al. Evaluation of feeding difficulties using videofluoroscopic swallow study and swallowing therapy in infants and children. Pediatrics & Neonatology 2023;64(5):547–53.
25. Martin-Harris B, Canon CL, Bonilha HS, et al. Best practices in modified barium swallow studies. Am J Speech Lang Pathol 2020;29(2S):1078–93.
26. Silva-Munhoz LdFd, Bühler KEB, Limongi SCO. Comparison between clinical and videofluoroscopic evaluation of swallowing in children with suspected dysphagia. CoDAS: SciELO Brasil; 2015. p. 186–92.

27. Maybee JL, Harrington BM, Prager JD. Pediatric Flexible Endoscopic Evaluation of Swallowing. Multidisciplinary Management of Pediatric Voice and Swallowing Disorders 2020;167–83.
28. Miller CK, Schroeder JW Jr, Langmore S. Fiberoptic Endoscopic Evaluation of Swallowing Across the Age Spectrum. Am J Speech Lang Pathol 2020;29(2s):967–78 (In eng).
29. Cerchiari A, Tofani M, Giordani C, et al. Development and Pilot Study of a Pediatric Screening for Feeding and Swallowing Disorders in Infants and Children: The Pediatric Screening–Priority Evaluation Dysphagia (PS–PED). Children 2023;10(4):638.
30. Zang J, Nienstedt JC, Koseki J-C, et al. Pediatric flexible endoscopic evaluation of swallowing: critical analysis of implementation and future perspectives. Dysphagia 2022;37(3):622–8.
31. Printza A, Sdravou K, Triaridis S. Dysphagia Management in Children: Implementation and Perspectives of Flexible Endoscopic Evaluation of Swallowing (FEES). Children 2022;9(12):1857.
32. Haller L, Osterbauer B, Maldonado K, et al. Factors impacting participation in flexible endoscopic evaluation of swallowing in children. Int J Pediatr Otorhinolaryngol 2020;138:110323 (In eng).
33. Martin-Harris B, Carson KA, Pinto JM, et al. BaByVFSSImP© a novel measurement tool for videofluoroscopic assessment of swallowing impairment in bottle-fed babies: establishing a standard. Dysphagia 2020;35:90–8.
34. Rosenbek JC, Robbins JA, Roecker EB, et al. A penetration-aspiration scale. Dysphagia 1996;11:93–8.
35. Stanley MA, Shepherd N, Duvall N, et al. Clinical identification of feeding and swallowing disorders in 0–6 month old infants with Down syndrome. Am J Med Genet 2019;179(2):177–82.
36. Simons JP, Greenberg LL, Mehta DK, et al. Laryngomalacia and swallowing function in children. Laryngoscope 2016;126(2):478–84 (In eng).
37. Scott BL, Lam D, MacArthur C. Laryngomalacia and swallow dysfunction. Ear. Nose & Throat Journal 2019;98(10):613–6.
38. Skoretz SA, Anger N, Wellman L, et al. A systematic review of tracheostomy modifications and swallowing in adults. Dysphagia 2020;35:935–47.
39. Streppel M, Veder LL, Pullens B, et al. Swallowing problems in children with a tracheostomy tube. Int J Pediatr Otorhinolaryngol 2019;124:30–3.
40. O'Connor LR, Morris NR, Paratz J. Physiological and clinical outcomes associated with use of one-way speaking valves on tracheostomised patients: A systematic review. Heart Lung 2019;48(4):356–64.
41. Zabih W, Holler T, Syed F, et al. The use of speaking valves in children with tracheostomy tubes. Respir Care 2017;62(12):1594–601.
42. Hill RR, Pados BF. Gastrointestinal Symptom Improvement for Infants Following Tongue-Tie Correction. Clin Pediatr (Phila) 2023;62(2):136–42 (In eng).
43. Geddes DT, Langton DB, Gollow I, et al. Frenulotomy for breastfeeding infants with ankyloglossia: effect on milk removal and sucking mechanism as imaged by ultrasound. Pediatrics 2008;122(1):e188–94 (In eng).
44. Shah S, Allen P, Walker R, et al. Upper Lip Tie: Anatomy, Effect on Breastfeeding, and Correlation With Ankyloglossia. Laryngoscope 2021;131(5):E1701–6 (In eng).

Assessing Dysphagia in the Adult

Laurence Gascon, MD, MSc, FRCSC[a,b,*], Paul C. Bryson, MD, MBA[a,b], Michael Benninger, MD[a,b], Martin B. Brodsky, PhD, MSc, CCC-SLP[a,b,c,d]

KEYWORDS

- Dysphagia • Assessment • Swallowing disorders • Swallowing evaluation
- Adult dysphagia • Deglutition • Deglutition disorders

KEY POINTS

- Dysphagia has a substantial impact on the quality of life for adults across diverse populations, including the elderly, individuals with neurological conditions, and those undergoing cancer treatments.
- Clinical and quality of life implications of dysphagia are significant and require thorough assessment. Assessment modalities for dysphagia in adults may include clinical history, physical examination, clinical evaluation, radiographic evaluation, endoscopic evaluation, and manometric evaluation.
- By combining various assessment methods, clinicians can achieve a comprehensive understanding of swallowing function, leading to targeted intervention strategies to enhance overall management.

Difficulty in swallowing, clinically termed *dysphagia*, profoundly affects the quality of life for millions worldwide, presenting challenges in various stages of the swallowing process. From oral preparation to safe transit past the airway, consequences of dysphagia include malnutrition, dehydration, aspiration pneumonia, and emotional distress.[1,2] This review delves into assessing adult swallowing function, emphasizing the importance of accurate methods for effective treatment.

EPIDEMIOLOGY

The impact of dysphagia spans diverse age groups and health conditions, with high prevalence among the elderly, particularly in long-term care facilities (30%–40% in

[a] Head and Neck Institute, Cleveland Clinic, Cleveland, OH, USA; [b] Cleveland Clinic Voice Center; [c] Department of Physical Medicine and Rehabilitation, Johns Hopkins University, Baltimore, MD, USA; [d] Division of Pulmonary and Critical Care Medicine, Johns Hopkins University, Baltimore, MD, USA
* Corresponding author. Cleveland Clinic Voice Center, Cleveland Clinic, 9500 Euclid Avenue, Cleveland, OH 44195.
E-mail address: gasconl@ccf.org

Otolaryngol Clin N Am 57 (2024) 523–530
https://doi.org/10.1016/j.otc.2024.03.003
0030-6665/24/© 2024 Elsevier Inc. All rights reserved.

those aged over 65 years).[3,4] Its presence in hospitalized adults correlates with extended stays, higher costs, post-acute facility discharges, and increased mortality.[5,6] Dysphagia is not exclusive to the elderly, arising as a secondary diagnosis in various conditions such as electrolyte imbalance, stroke, pneumonia, and cardiac diseases.[6] Dysphagia can also affect individuals undergoing head and neck cancer treatments, those with congenital anomalies, and those with degenerative conditions.[1,7] Its dynamic nature and varying severity necessitate tailored treatments, possibly including any combination of changes to food consistencies, nonoral feedings, postural adjustments, and exercises.[8,9]

The prevalence of dysphagia in different populations underscores the need for vigilant surveillance and comprehensive assessment methods. Despite its significant impact, dysphagia is often underdiagnosed, hindering timely intervention.[10] This article emphasizes the importance of sophisticated assessment techniques for early detection and tailored interventions, aiming to enhance the overall quality of life for individuals affected by dysphagia.

INITIAL ASSESSMENT AND PHYSICAL EXAMINATION
Clinical History

Swallowing tests fall into clinical and instrumental categories. Clinical assessments commence with a comprehensive medical history, gathering information through patient reports, validated questionnaires, or clinician-initiated interviews.[4,11] Questionnaires targeting general symptoms and impact on quality of life, sometimes specific to patient populations, offer valuable insights.[12–14]

Patient history review includes recent illnesses, conditions, hospital visits, laboratories, medications, radiologic evaluations, and nursing notes. Neurologic and pulmonary conditions, autoimmune issues, past radiotherapy, head and neck malignancy, and surgical history, especially involving the head, neck, or esophagus, are crucial. Patients often report sensations such as food sticking, odynophagia, coughing, or general swallowing difficulty. Changes in eating habits, problematic foods, and regurgitation of solids indicate potential issues such as diverticulum or reflux.[15] Clinical signs such as pneumonia, voice changes, breathing difficulties, or frequent throat clearing signal a possible dysphagia and aspiration, the understanding of which aids diagnosis. Causes may involve neuromuscular issues, with more severe symptoms potentially with liquids, or mechanical factors such as osteophytes, diverticula, tumors, or webs.[16]

Differentiating difficulty with solids and liquids is crucial. Solid challenges may indicate structural lesions such as tumors, webs, or strictures in the esophagus. Liquid difficulties may suggest motility disorders like scleroderma or achalasia, though not mutually exclusive. A history of esophageal obstruction, particularly in younger adults, may hint at conditions like eosinophilic esophagitis.[17]

Physical Examination

In adult dysphagia assessment, a thorough head and neck examination is indispensable, encompassing a comprehensive evaluation of anatomy and all cranial nerves. The oral cavity examination includes assessing mucosal integrity, soft palate and tongue movement, and dentition. Patients should be queried about taste and sensation alterations, and dentition and denture fit are also scrutinized. Neck palpation identifies masses and tension, while laryngeal elevation during swallowing is observed. Boyce's sign, indicative of Zenker's diverticulum, may manifest as a gurgling sound upon neck pressure.[18]

Flexible laryngoscopy offers detailed mucosal and anatomic assessment, crucial for swallowing evaluation. The initial examination focuses on soft palate movement, detecting velopharyngeal insufficiency, and nasal regurgitation.[19] Saliva pooling in valleculae and pyriform sinuses strongly suggests dysphagia. Attention to masses or asymmetries throughout the examination is required.[20] Pharyngeal contractions, vocal fold movements, and laryngeal reflexes are observed.[21] The tidal wave sign, indicating esophageal inlet backflow, suggests diverticulum presence.

Transnasal Esophagoscopy

Transnasal esophagoscopy (TNE) is a novel technique for dysphagia assessment in adults. This minimally invasive procedure offers a direct, real-time view of the esophagus through a slender, flexible endoscope inserted via the nasal passage, eliminating the need for sedation. TNE's high-resolution imaging capabilities enable detailed examination of mucosal surfaces, facilitating the detection of anatomic abnormalities, inflammation, and foreign bodies.[22] Biopsies can also be performed for comprehensive diagnostic assessment.[23] With its dynamic assessment capabilities, TNE allows clinicians to observe swallowing function and detect transit abnormalities. While TNE excels in visualizing mucosa, its focus on the luminal aspect limits the deep tissue layer assessment. Nonetheless, its advantages in patient acceptability and convenience make it a valuable tool in comprehensive dysphagia evaluation.

Clinical Swallowing Evaluation

A clinical swallowing evaluation (CSE) offers a noninvasive method for assessing swallow function in adults and is performed by speech–language pathologists (SLPs) who observe swallowing dynamics and note any abnormalities or difficulties. SLPs evaluate the patient's response to different food and liquid consistencies, noting signs of penetration or aspiration such as coughing, throat clearing, or a wet, gurgly voice. The 3 oz water swallow test was identified as the best predictive value in ruling out aspiration.[24,25] While lacking the precision of instrumental assessments, the CSE provides immediate and cost-effective insights into swallowing function through behavioral response, though it may not detect silent aspiration or specific anatomic abnormalities. It allows for real-time observation of the patient's neuromuscular integrity and cognitive functions.[26]

DIAGNOSTIC AND INSTRUMENTAL STUDIES

Instrumental evaluations of swallowing offer detailed insights into swallowing anatomy and function, addressing physiologic aspects such as timing, strength, and coordination. These assessments guide plans for nutritional intake, rehabilitation, and additional consultations by identifying causes of dysfunction rather than identifying clinical signs through noninstrumental screenings and assessments. Results are not binary and should not be viewed as "pass/fail."[27] Major findings include identifying the cause of airway invasion, distinguishing between laryngeal penetration and aspiration, and offering strategies to maintain airway safety during swallowing.

Esophagram/Barium Swallow

The esophagram, or barium swallow study, is an important diagnostic tool in instrumental swallowing assessments for adults. This radiographic procedure employs videofluoroscopy to provide dynamic imaging of the swallowing process, offering detailed insights into upper gastrointestinal tract anatomy and function from the pharynx and upper esophageal sphincter (cricopharyngeus) through the lower esophageal sphincter (ie, gastroesophageal junction) and into the stomach. Through the administration of liquid barium contrast, clinicians gain the ability to visualize and analyze the passage of liquids through the esophagus, allowing for an evaluation of esophageal swallowing function and the detection of underlying structural abnormalities or functional impairments. The primary objective of the examination is to identify disordered anatomy and/or bolus movement during swallowing, facilitated by both anterior–posterior and lateral views for real-time visualization. Notably, the barium swallow is adept at detecting structural abnormalities such as strictures, diverticula, and tumors.[28] However, caution is required to promptly discontinue the examination if aspiration is observed. Limitations include potential aversion to barium ingestion, radiation exposure concerns, and gastrointestinal discomfort. The success of the examination is contingent on patient cooperation, which may pose challenges in individuals with cognitive and/or behavioral issues.

Videofluoroscopic Swallow Study/Modified Barium Swallow Study

The modified barium swallow study (MBSS), one of the 2 gold standards for instrumental swallowing evaluation, is a videofluoroscopic technique collaboratively performed by a SLP and radiology clinicians.[29] It provides a real-time assessment of oropharyngeal swallow and esophageal clearance, identifying underlying physiology contributing to dysphagia. Standardized protocols such as the Modified Barium Swallow Impairment Profile facilitate detailed evaluation using Varibar barium consistencies at standard volumes and a standard frame rate of 30 frames per second.[30]

The MBSS enables real-time observation of the patient's response to swallowing maneuvers and compensatory strategies for improved bolus clearance and airway safety, aiding in prognosis for dysphagia rehabilitation and recovery.[31] While offering a thorough examination, it is important to note that the MBSS has limitations, such as the inability to directly assess saliva control/containment, the use of nonfood items (ie, barium), and exposure to ionizing radiation. The MBSS remains a low-dose radiation examination, ensuring safety through shielding and adherence to safety protocols.[32] It remains an indispensable tool for understanding swallowing function in adults and allows for the observation of therapeutic strategies and swallowing maneuvers contributing to improved safety, health, and quality of life for patients with dysphagia.[31,33]

Flexible Endoscopic Evaluation of Swallowing

Flexible endoscopic evaluation of swallowing (FEES), the second of 2 gold standards for instrumental swallowing evaluation, is typically conducted by SLPs and otolaryngologists.[27] The evaluation begins with a laryngeal examination, focusing on pharyngeal and laryngeal anatomy and function, including soft palate closure, pharyngeal symmetry, presence of secretions and their location, base of tongue movement, phonation, and pharyngeal contraction. Subsequently, various food and drink consistencies are tested, allowing assessment of passive bolus overflow, pharyngeal coating or stasis, penetration, aspiration, post-swallow residue, backflow from the esophagus, effectiveness of protective mechanisms like coughing or throat clearing, and instances of double swallows.

FEES utilizes standard food and drinks for a practical evaluation of swallowing, with outpatients encouraged to bring problematic foods for assessment. It allows for immediate and direct visualization of the anatomy and physiology of swallowing. Like MBSS, FEES serves as both a diagnostic and therapeutic modality for compensatory techniques, and its portability allows for use in various settings, including outpatient and home environments. Moreover, the procedure can be repeated as needed, allowing for ongoing monitoring of changes in swallowing function and the effectiveness of interventions. However, limitations include patient discomfort during nasopharyngeal insertion and a focus on the pharyngeal phase with limited views of the oral and esophageal phases. Finally, rare complications have been reported such as epistaxis, mucosal perforation, vasovagal reactions, and the remote chance of laryngospasm.[34]

Manometry

Manometry is a valuable tool for assessing dysphagia in adults, offering insights into pharyngeal and esophageal function and motility. Unlike MBSS and FEES, which visualize anatomy, manometry measures muscular contractions and pressure changes during swallowing using pressure sensors along its length.[35,36] Standard esophageal manometry spans from the cricopharyngeus to the gastroesophageal junction. High-resolution manometry allows contraction of the pharynx to be measured as well, with sensors that extend from the hypopharynx through the gastroesophageal junction.[37]

Upper esophageal sphincter pathologies can be assessed with manometry.[37,38] This region is, however, found to be dependent on the volumes of the swallow bolus, which may be inadequately represented during manometry. It is the best modality to assess motility and lower esophageal sphincter dysfunction.[39] Manometry aids in identifying conditions that may contribute to dysphagia, including conditions such as esophageal spasms and ineffective esophageal motility.[40] The assessment provides detailed information to guide targeted treatment strategies. Although manometry may cause discomfort, it is generally well tolerated and safe, playing a crucial role in the comprehensive evaluation of dysphagia in adults.

pH Testing

pH testing can provide guidance in otherwise negative dysphagia workup in special populations such as young adults or postgastrectomy patients. Results can signal referral for gastroenterology, surgical fundoplication, or mucosal ablation.

pH testing provides information about the frequency and severity of gastroesophageal reflux disease (GERD)".[41] It involves placing a pH probe into the esophagus to measure acid levels over a period of time, typically 24 hours; however, in-office pH testing tools are available for otolaryngologists to place in the office and interpret.

SUMMARY

The comprehensive assessment of swallowing function in adult patients necessitates a multifaceted approach integrating various modalities. Clinical evaluation and physical examination lay the foundation and provide crucial insights into symptoms and potential causes. Videofluoroscopy and esophagram offer real-time radiographic assessments, allowing for detection of anatomic abnormalities from lips to stomach. FEES provides real-time visualization of the pharyngeal phase of swallowing and a highly sensitive view of the pharynx and larynx, while TNE provides high-resolution mucosal visualization of the esophagus. Manometry, with or without pH testing, offers sensitive pressure measurements to identify motility disorders. By judiciously employing this array of modalities among a group of multidisciplinary, well-trained clinicians, a well-rounded understanding of swallowing function will lead to a precise diagnosis with personalized intervention strategies for the overall management of adults grappling with dysphagia.

CLINICS CARE POINTS

- Dysphagia can lead to severe consequences such as malnutrition, dehydration, aspiration pneumonia, and even death.
- Indicators of dysphagia to be vigilant for include weight loss, pneumonia, voice changes while eating/swallowing, breathing difficulties, and frequent throat clearing.
- Flexible laryngoscopy and TNE offer safe, minimally invasive, and well-tolerated visualization of pharyngeal, laryngeal, and esophageal dynamics.
- The 3 oz water swallow test is the best predictive screening for aspiration.
- The MBSS assesses all phases of swallowing using barium and provides diagnostic, nonbinary results.
- Manometry is ideal for assessing esophageal motility, pressures, and lower esophageal sphincter compliance, while pH testing evaluates GERD severity and frequency.
- Collaborative swallowing assessment such as videofluoroscopic swallow study and FEES provides real-time, dynamic visualization of swallowing, mirroring real-world eating conditions and enhancing clinical relevance.

DISCLOSURE

The authors have no financial or commercial conflicts of interests.

REFERENCES

1. Krebbers I, Pilz W, Vanbelle S, et al. Affective Symptoms and Oropharyngeal Dysphagia in Head-and-Neck Cancer Patients: A Systematic Review. Dysphagia 2023;38(1):127–44.
2. Baijens LW, Clave P, Cras P, et al. European Society for Swallowing Disorders - European Union Geriatric Medicine Society white paper: oropharyngeal dysphagia as a geriatric syndrome. Clin Interv Aging 2016;11:1403–28.
3. Keller H, Vucea V, Slaughter SE, et al. Prevalence of Malnutrition or Risk in Residents in Long Term Care: Comparison of Four Tools. J Nutr Gerontol Geriatr 2019;38(4):329–44.
4. Sari DW, Aurizki GE, Indarwati R, et al. The Provision of Texture-Modified Foods in Long-term Care Facilities by Health Professionals: Protocol for a Scoping Review. JMIR Res Protoc 2023;12:e44201.
5. Patel DA, Krishnaswami S, Steger E, et al. Economic and survival burden of dysphagia among inpatients in the United States. Dis Esophagus 2018;31(1):1–7.
6. Altman KW, Yu GP, Schaefer SD. Consequence of dysphagia in the hospitalized patient: impact on prognosis and hospital resources. Arch Otolaryngol Head Neck Surg 2010;136(8):784–9.
7. Moore KA, Ford PJ, Farah CS. Support needs and quality of life in oral cancer: a systematic review. Int J Dent Hyg 2014;12(1):36–47.
8. McCabe D, Ashford J, Wheeler-Hegland K, et al. Evidence-based systematic review: Oropharyngeal dysphagia behavioral treatments. Part IV–impact of dysphagia treatment on individuals' postcancer treatments. J Rehabil Res Dev 2009;46(2):205–14.
9. Wheeler-Hegland K, Frymark T, Schooling T, et al. Evidence-based systematic review: Oropharyngeal dysphagia behavioral treatments. Part V--applications for clinicians and researchers. J Rehabil Res Dev 2009;46(2):215–22.

10. Gonzalez-Fernandez M, Gardyn M, Wyckoff S, et al. Validation of ICD-9 Code 787.2 for identification of individuals with dysphagia from administrative databases. Dysphagia 2009;24(4):398–402.
11. Paris G, Martinaud O, Hannequin D, et al. Clinical screening of oropharyngeal dysphagia in patients with ALS. Ann Phys Rehabil Med 2012;55(9–10):601–8.
12. Chen AY, Frankowski R, Bishop-Leone J, et al. The development and validation of a dysphagia-specific quality-of-life questionnaire for patients with head and neck cancer: the M. D. Anderson dysphagia inventory. Arch Otolaryngol Head Neck Surg 2001;127(7):870–6.
13. Kim DY, Park HS, Park SW, et al. The impact of dysphagia on quality of life in stroke patients. Medicine (Baltim) 2020;99(34):e21795.
14. Diamanti L, Borrelli P, Dubbioso R, et al, DYALS Study Group. Validation of the DYALS (dysphagia in amyotrophic lateral sclerosis) questionnaire for the evaluation of dysphagia in ALS patients. Neurol Sci 2022;43(5):3195–200.
15. Hendrix TR. Art and science of history taking in the patient with difficulty swallowing. Dysphagia 1993;8(2):69–73.
16. O'Horo JC, Rogus-Pulia N, Garcia-Arguello L, et al. Bedside diagnosis of dysphagia: a systematic review. J Hosp Med 2015;10(4):256–65.
17. Benninger MS, Strohl M, Holy CE, et al. Prevalence of atopic disease in patients with eosinophilic esophagitis. Int Forum Allergy Rhinol 2017;7(8):757–62.
18. Sharma SC, Sakthivel P, Singh S, et al. Boyce's sign in a large Zenker's diverticulum. Lancet Gastroenterol Hepatol 2019;4(9):742.
19. Langmore SE, Scarborough DR, Kelchner LN, et al. Tutorial on Clinical Practice for Use of the Fiberoptic Endoscopic Evaluation of Swallowing Procedure With Adult Populations: Part 1. Am J Speech Lang Pathol 2022;31(1):163–87.
20. Hunting A, Steffanoni B, Jacques A, et al. Accumulated Secretions and Associated Aerodigestive Function in Patients With Dysphagia. Am J Speech Lang Pathol 2023;32(6):2691–702.
21. Kaneoka A, Pisegna JM, Inokuchi H, et al. Relationship Between Laryngeal Sensory Deficits, Aspiration, and Pneumonia in Patients with Dysphagia. Dysphagia 2018;33(2):192–9.
22. Belafsky PC, Postma GN, Daniel E, et al. Transnasal esophagoscopy. Otolaryngology–head and neck surgery 2001;125(6):588–9.
23. Postma GN, Cohen JT, Belafsky PC, et al. Transnasal esophagoscopy: revisited (over 700 consecutive cases). Laryngoscope 2005;115(2):321–3.
24. Brodsky MB, Suiter DM, Gonzalez-Fernandez M, et al. Screening Accuracy for Aspiration Using Bedside Water Swallow Tests: A Systematic Review and Meta-Analysis. Chest 2016;150(1):148–63.
25. Suiter DM, Leder SB. Clinical utility of the 3-ounce water swallow test. Dysphagia 2008;23(3):244–50.
26. Carnaby-Mann G, Lenius K. The bedside examination in dysphagia. Phys Med Rehabil Clin N Am 2008;19(4):747–68.
27. Langmore SE. History of Fiberoptic Endoscopic Evaluation of Swallowing for Evaluation and Management of Pharyngeal Dysphagia: Changes over the Years. Dysphagia 2017;32(1):27–38.
28. Wilkinson JM, Codipilly DC, Wilfahrt RP. Dysphagia: Evaluation and Collaborative Management. Am Fam Physician 2021;103(2):97–106.
29. Aviv JE. Prospective, randomized outcome study of endoscopy versus modified barium swallow in patients with dysphagia. Laryngoscope 2000;110(4):563–74.

30. Mulheren RW, Azola A, Gonzalez-Fernandez M. Do Ratings of Swallowing Function Differ by Videofluoroscopic Rate? An Exploratory Analysis in Patients After Acute Stroke. Arch Phys Med Rehabil 2019;100(6):1085–90.
31. Martin-Harris B, Brodsky MB, Michel Y, et al. MBS measurement tool for swallow impairment–MBSImp: establishing a standard. Dysphagia 2008;23(4):392–405.
32. Bonilha HS, Wilmskoetter J, Tipnis S, et al. Relationships Between Radiation Exposure Dose, Time, and Projection in Videofluoroscopic Swallowing Studies. Am J Speech Lang Pathol 2019;28(3):1053–9.
33. Hazelwood RJ, Armeson KE, Hill EG, et al. Identification of Swallowing Tasks From a Modified Barium Swallow Study That Optimize the Detection of Physiological Impairment. J Speech Lang Hear Res 2017;60(7):1855–63.
34. Dziewas R, Damm-Lunau R, Dunkel J, et al. Safety and clinical impact of FEES - results of the FEES-registry. Neurol Res Pract 2019;1:16.
35. Ott DJ, Richter JE, Chen YM, et al. Esophageal radiography and manometry: correlation in 172 patients with dysphagia. AJR Am J Roentgenol 1987;149(2): 307–11.
36. Moretz WH 3rd, Postma GN, Burkhead LM, et al. High-resolution esophageal manometry. Ear Nose Throat J 2006;85(2):85.
37. Jones CA, Ciucci MR, Hammer MJ, et al. A multisensor approach to improve manometric analysis of the upper esophageal sphincter. Laryngoscope 2016; 126(3):657–64.
38. Norton P, Herbella FAM, Schlottmann F, et al. The upper esophageal sphincter in the high-resolution manometry era. Langenbeck's Arch Surg 2021;406(8): 2611–9.
39. Yadlapati R, Kahrilas PJ, Fox MR, et al. Esophageal motility disorders on high-resolution manometry: Chicago classification version 4.0((c)). Neuro Gastroenterol Motil 2021;33(1):e14058.
40. Agrawal A, Hila A, Tutuian R, et al. Manometry and impedance characteristics of achalasia. Facts and myths. J Clin Gastroenterol 2008;42(3):266–70.
41. Mari A, Sweis R. Assessment and management of dysphagia and achalasia. Clin Med 2021;21(2):119–23.

Pediatric Dysphagia

Wade McClain, DO[a],*, Jordan Luttrell, MD[b], Elton Lambert, MD[c]

KEYWORDS

- Dysphagia • Oropharyngeal • Deglutition • Aspiration pneumonia
- Congenital abnormalities

KEY POINTS

- Pediatric dysphagia is a commonly diagnosed condition associated with many congenital and acquired conditions.
- Normal physiologic swallow is a complex sequence of actions that can be disrupted at many points during the process.
- Timely identification and management of dysphagia is important to avoid serious and preventable sequelae.
- Nonsurgical management of dysphagia including medical and practical treatments can be used to address the condition.

Swallowing is the process by which food, liquid, saliva, and pharyngeal secretions are transferred from the oral cavity and the pharynx to the esophagus and the stomach. Normal swallowing in children is necessary for adequate oral nutrition, airway protection, and contributes to quality of life and bonding in the family unit.[1] Dysphagia is any interruption of normal swallowing and has significant impact on children and their families.

Swallowing can be divided into the oral preparatory, oral transit, and pharyngeal and esophageal phases. Dysphagia is classified by the phase that it occurs. The oral preparatory phase involves the introduction of food and liquid into the oral cavity by the expression of fluid from a bottle, nipple/other drinking vessel and solids with utensils (including hands). Lip seal, tongue elevation, and mastication coordinate to form and control a bolus mixed with saliva that is propelled to the pharynx during the oral transit phase.[2,3] The soft palate elevates, closing off the nasopharynx to prevent velopharyngeal reflux. Oral transit time is typically less than a second,[4] and a prolonged oral transit time may indicate oral phase dysphagia associated with neurologic conditions.[5]

[a] Department of Otolaryngology/Head and Neck Surgery, University of North Carolina, 101 Manning Drive Campus, Box #7070, Chapel Hill, NC 27514, USA; [b] Department of Otolaryngology, University of Tennessee Health Science Center, 910 Madison Avenue, Suite 430, Memphis, TN 38163, USA; [c] Department of Otolaryngology, Baylor College of Medicine, Texas Children's Hospital, 6701 Fannin Street, MC:CC640, Houston, TX 77030, USA
* Corresponding author. University of North Carolina, Department of Otolaryngology/Head and Neck Surgery, 101 Manning Drive Campus, Box #7070, Chapel Hill, NC 27514.
E-mail address: Wade.mcclain@gmail.com

Otolaryngol Clin N Am 57 (2024) 531–540
https://doi.org/10.1016/j.otc.2024.02.010
0030-6665/24/© 2024 Elsevier Inc. All rights reserved.

During a normal pharyngeal phase, the bolus is propelled through the pharynx to the esophagus, while protecting the airway from aspiration. This requires coordination among velopharyngeal closure, hyoid elevation, tongue base retraction, pharyngeal constrictor contraction, laryngeal elevation, epiglottic retroflexion, true and false vocal fold adduction, and cricopharyngeal opening. Pharyngeal transit time is less than 0.5 seconds.[4] The esophageal phase begins as the cricopharyngeus opens, and the bolus advances via peristalsis to the stomach.

Food and liquid bolus require effective management for nutrition, but secretion management is of great importance. Saliva from the oral cavity, and pharyngeal secretions consisting of nasal and tracheobronchial tree mucous; and regurgitated esophageal and gastric contents must be swallowed effectively to prevent pulmonary sequelae of aspiration.

Swallowing occurs through both voluntary and involuntary mechanisms controlled through centers in the brainstem such as the nucleus tractus solitarus modulated by cortical swallowing centers. The oral preparatory and transit phases are mediated by sensory afferents of cranial nerve (CN) V, and motor efferents of CN V, VII, and XII, and is mostly voluntary. The pharyngeal phase is voluntary and involuntary with sensory input from CN V, IX, and X and motor from CN V, IX, X, and IX, while the esophageal phase is mostly involuntary with sensory and motor control by CN X.[6]

Coordination of phases of swallowing requires organization of the anatomic sites, sensory and motor inputs to allow for safe transfer of bolus from the oral cavity to the esophagus. Increase in transit times, delays in initiation of the phases of swallowing and decreases in the frequencies of swallowing can lead to dysphagia. Transit time from the oral cavity to the cricopharyngeal is 0.44 to 2 seconds in infants and toddlers.[4] Transit times vary based on consistency of food and liquid, vessels, and flow rate.[4,7] Spontaneous swallowing occurs about once per minute in children without neurologic conditions and are reduced in children with cerebral palsy.[8] For safe swallowing, laryngeal closure during the pharyngeal phase should occur at the end of the oral transit phase. Variability in the initiation of the pharyngeal phase contributes to dysphagia. Bolus arrival to oropharynx prior to start of the pharyngeal phase may increase aspiration risk.

Airway protection during swallow requires coordination of the swallow–breathing reflex and in infants the suck–swallow–breathe reflex. A normal ratio of suck: swallow: breathe is 1:1:1 or 2:2:1 in infants.[9] Additionally, ventilation rate decreases during bottle feeding inversely with swallow frequency.[10] Neural connections between the brainstem swallow centers and respiratory centers mediate the function and development of the swallow–breathe reflex,[11] and it is the maturation of these centers that contribute to the normal development of swallowing in children.

DEVELOPMENT OF SWALLOWING

Fetal swallowing has been observed through ultrasonography and plays an important role in amniotic fluid regulation. Fetal suckling responses can be seen as early as 15 weeks with consistent swallowing seen at 24 weeks.[12] Progression to term as evidenced by patterns in premature infants is marked with improved oral motor coordination. Anterior–posterior movement of the tongue leads to rhythmic peristaltic waves that propels liquid to the oropharynx, which is coordinated with soft palate elevation.[13] In the pharyngeal and esophageal phase increased pharyngeal propulsion and a decrease in relaxation time of the upper esophageal sphincter (UES) occur as premature infants mature. Premature infants aged less than 34 weeks have neural immaturity that impairs safe swallow coordination.[14] Non-nutritive suckling and swallowing exercises improve coordination in all phases of swallowing.[15]

The development of swallowing in healthy term and premature infants progresses with the maturation of their anatomy and physiology. At term, the mandible is disproportionately small, and the tongue fills the oral cavity with little room for movement. The epiglottis contacts the soft palate resulting in a proportionately smaller pharyngal volume. In the first 6 months of life, the oral cavity enlarges, the mandible grows, and the larynx descends. This leads to improved tongue mobility from an anterior–posterior dominant pattern associated with suckling to more complex movement patterns, and improved pharyngeal propulsion.[16] Head, jaw, and trunk control improve in the first 6 months and is key to safe swallowing.[17] These developmental milestones allow for the safe introduction of solids, the use of utensils, and the use of alternative vessels for liquids besides bottles.

The development of lip closure, tongue movement, jaw development, and tooth eruption progress from infant through the early childhood stage leading to the introduction of more complex solids as chewing, bolus formation, and propulsion matures. Guiding children through this development also requires the introduction of foods and liquids varying textures and tastes that are safe for their developmental stage. Effective chewing habits are not only dependent on the appearance of the 1st and 2nd molars (eruption from 1.5–3 years), but also bite force and bolus handling. Chewing efficiency (thus decreasing aspiration risk with solids) optimizes between the age of 3 and 5 years.[18] The AAP recommends the introduction of solids that pose a choking hazard, such as nuts, after the age of 4 years.[19] Swallow development continues with soft tissue, skeletal and neuronal maturation through adulthood. Disturbances in development of swallow can lead to dysphagia and the associated sequalae.

PRESENTATION AND SEQUALAE OF DYSPHAGIA

Children with dysphagia classically present with coughing or choking on food or liquids. Subtle signs of dysphagia include drooling, prolonged feeding, decreased swallowing frequency, and oral aversion. Chronic cough and recurrent respiratory infections may be one of the first signs of dysphagia in "silent" aspiration, when no obvious symptoms occur during swallowing.

Dysphagia in children causes significant effects on nutrition, quality of life, and respiratory health. Interventions for dysphagia such as changes in nipple size, feeding vessels, and thickening and placement of enteral feeding tubes must take nutrition into account. Dysphagia can be factor for poor weight gain in children.[20] Health-related quality of life is reduced in patients with dysphagia.[21–23] Parental worry about a child's health and feeding, and the emotional impact on daily activities is contributor to reduced quality of life for families of children with dysphagia. Home care for dysphagia such as thickening liquids have observed benefits for families, but the frustrations experienced by families must be acknowledged.[24] Families with a child with feeding difficulties are also more likely to have a caregiver leave a job and experience food insufficiency,[25] and so the impact of pediatric dysphagia on the family unit should not be understated.

Dysphagia can have significant effects on respiratory health and associated health-related quality of life. Dysphagia and aspiration can lead to a whole host of respiratory complications including chronic cough, recurrent respiratory infections, aspiration pneumonia, and need for bronchodilators/inhaled steroids. More serious consequences of aspiration include chronic lung disease, bronchiectasis, and chronic respiratory failure. Controversies lie in whether these sequalae of aspiration are due to aspiration of food or saliva.[26] Regardless of the underlying pathophysiology, practitioners must be aware of the potential respiratory morbidity in patients with dysphagia and who is at most risk. Patients with laryngeal penetration or aspiration on a swallow study have an increased risk of aspiration pneumonia regardless of presenting symptoms.[27,28] In children with chronic conditions such as cerebral palsy, dysphagia increases the risk of pulmonary complications.[29,30]

Children with dysphagia have increased health care utilization and costs,[25] especially when there is associated respiratory morbidity. Inpatient and outpatient costs are increased in patients with dysphagia due to increased hospitalizations, tests, treatment, and therapy. Care pathways and multidisciplinary care may decrease these costs.[31]

EPIDEMIOLOGY

Pediatric dysphagia has been estimated to impact about 1% of the general pediatric population based on large scale survey responses to the Centers for Disease Control (CDC).[32,33] In certain high-risk populations such as children with gastrointestinal (GI) disease, respiratory disease, and developmental delay, dysphagia is thought to impact anywhere from 5% to 99% of patients depending on the severity of the associated comorbidity.[34–38] However, estimating the true prevalence is challenging as surveys may underestimate the true disease burden.[33] A large-scale epidemiologic study of dysphagia in children has not been performed as of this writing. Published estimates of incidence has a high degree of variability due to the natural sampling and publication bias related to the study of specific populations. There is likely an overall increase in incidence due to improved survival of premature infants and medically fragile children as well as improved efforts at surveillance.[39,40] Lastly, there is inherent challenge in accurate diagnosis due to efforts to minimize radiation exposure, difficulty with patient participation, variability in trained assessment, and accuracy of parental report.[41–44]

ETIOLOGY

Feeding and swallowing are complex activities that begin development in utero and continue throughout infancy and childhood with both voluntary and involuntary components as detailed earlier. Abnormal structural, neurocognitive, muscular, or psychosocial development can lead to difficulty with single or multiple components of the process of swallowing. The etiology of dysphagia is often multifactorial (**Box 1**) and its identification can provide valuable information for prognosis and long-term treatment considerations.

Structural causes of dysphagia can broadly be divided into craniofacial abnormalities and esophageal/respiratory-related conditions. Craniofacial abnormalities can be recognized early in fetal screening/infancy and manifest as disruption in the negative pressure seal or with respiratory difficulty during feeding. These include cleft lip, cleft palate, severe ankyloglossia, and mandibular hypoplasia. Obstructive adenotonsillar hypertrophy can arise later in childhood and can contribute to dysphagia. Respiratory-esophageal conditions include choanal atresia, pyriform aperture stenosis, trachea–esophageal fistulae, laryngeal cleft, and laryngomalacia. Vascular anomalies and congenital heart defects can cause extrinsic compression of the aerodigestive tract contributing to dysphagia. While many of these are identified early in the neonatal period some of the more dynamic conditions can have less conspicuous presentations and present with poor weight gain, respiratory distress during feeding attempts, or cough/choking following a feeding attempt.

Another broad etiologic category of pediatric dysphagia includes neurocognitive and muscular dysfunction. These can present in central nervous system disorders

---

Box 1
Conditions commonly associated with pediatric dysphagia

Prematurity

Cerebral palsy

Intraventricular hemorrhage

Seizure disorders

Congenital infections

Congenital/acquired vocal cord paralysis/immobility

Gastroesophageal reflux disease

Eosinophilic esophagitis

Congenital cardiac disease

Vascular ring

Choanal atresia

Adenoid hypertrophy

Micro/retrognathia

Macroglossia

Vallecular cyst

Laryngomalacia

Laryngotracheal cleft

Subglottic stenosis

Tracheoesophageal fistula

Esophageal atresia

---

such as cerebral palsy, global developmental delay, neonatal brain injury, or chromosomal abnormalities often with poor initiation, inadequate coordination, and incomplete secretion management. Other cases can present with hypotonic muscle function that reduces the ability to produce and complete swallow of bolus. These can be present at birth in syndromic cases or develop during childhood in degenerative diseases. Both congenital and progressive cases tend to present with systemic coordination and functional concerns in addition to dysphagia. In contrast, peripheral nerve deficits such as cranial nerve paralysis, vocal cord hypofunction, and UES dysmotility tend to cause localized dysphagia or upper respiratory issues.

Psychosocial factors play a major role in dysphagia but should be considered distinctly from structural dysphagia. This includes primary oral aversion that arises due to limited early oral intake or trained behavior as a child develops. Secondary dysphagia can also occur due to a traumatic event such as severe illness or choking. It is crucial to consider the interplay between a child's psychiatric baseline with potential functional or communication issues manifesting as dysphagia. Other physiologic causes should always be ruled out prior to sole treatment of a functional issue.

COMORBIDITIES

A complete list of comorbidities associated with dysphagia is beyond the scope of this study; however, several conditions are highly associated with dysphagia in the pediatric population (see **Box 1**).[45] The most associated conditions with dysphagia are neurologic dysfunction or neurodevelopmental delay. The suck–swallow reflex in infancy and complete swallow response of childhood require highly complex neurologic integration that can be lacking in these conditions. It is estimated that 19.2% to 99% of cerebral palsy patients struggle with dysphagia with rates increasing with the severity of disease. Patients with communication disorders or autism spectrum disorder have been reported to have 4 to 15 times elevated risk of dysphagia.[46,47] Other neurologic disorders such as brain tumors, hydrocephalus, and seizures have also been shown to elevate the risk.[48]

Congenital heart disease is also commonly associated with dysphagia with 30% to 40% of patients experiencing aspiration and feeding difficulties respectively. This has been related to increased respiratory effort, higher rates of fatigue, persistent hypoxic states, and elevated metabolic requirements. Vocal cord dysfunction or paralysis which can commonly occur following cardiac procedures leads to higher rates of dysphagia.[49]

Several GI conditions can present with oropharyngeal dysphagia. Presenting symptoms are often similar and can be clinically difficult to differentiate what proportion is related to upper versus lower GI symptoms. The presence of gastroesophageal reflux disease (GERD) likely worsens oropharyngeal dysphagia by creating a hyperinflammatory state and higher risk of aspiration. Some studies have suggested that 90% or more of patients presenting with GERD also have concomitant dysphagia.[50,51] Severe conditions such as trachea–esophageal fistula or congenital diaphragmatic hernia completely inhibit normal swallow, whereas other dysmotility conditions, esophagitis, or food intolerance should be considered as contributing factors.

MEDICAL TREATMENT

The goals of treatment in dysphagia are to protect the airway, maintain hydration, meet nutritional goals, and facilitate normal development. Medical management is generally attempted in lower risk populations while surgical treatment is reserved for those with refractory or severe symptoms and is covered in detail elsewhere in this issue. As with most pediatric conditions, identifying the underlying cause is essential in choosing the correct treatment. Additionally, it is important to remember that the natural course of the disease in many patients is for an improvement in swallow function as the child develops.

First-line conservative treatment involves referral for speech/swallow evaluation and potential therapy. Speech therapists, occupational therapists, or certified lactation consultants are important members of the treatment team and can help guide initial intervention. Depending on the age of the child, positioning techniques can be employed to improve swallow. Neonates and infants can improve with varying nipple types and flow rates for bottle feeding or with nipple shields or paced feeding in breastfeeding.[20] Infants then transition to seated feeding with postural changes such as chin tuck, trunk/neck support, and variable utensils which can improve their overall feeding efficiency. Occasionally, a dietician may need to be incorporated into the care team to help optimize formula choice and rule out other dietary contributions to dysphagia.[52]

Another commonly employed treatment technique is texture modification or additive thickeners. Addition of thickener to liquid feedings changes the swallow mechanics and increases transit time and sensory input for better bolus handling. One advantage is that thickener can be titrated during swallow assessment to allow individualized patient care. Recent systematic review demonstrated that thickener use likely decreases the risk of penetration/aspiration; however, use of thickeners is not without risk as this also increases the risk of pharyngeal residue and possible aspiration of the thickened liquid.[53] Addition of thickener requires more oropharyngeal muscle strength for propulsion which potentiates a need for higher energy expenditure during feeding.[54] There are also implications regarding GI mobility, sensitivity/intolerance, and caloric changes to be considered. Overall, there is still a lack of high-quality empiric evidence or consensus guidelines on use of thickener but has potential benefit under close management of physician/speech therapy team.[55]

Management of concomitant reflux is an important treatment consideration. Recently published Pediatric Gastroesophageal Reflux Clinical Practice Guidelines recommend a 4 to 8 week trial of histamine blockade (H2BA) or proton pump inhibitor (PPI) for patients with clinical signs of GERD (back arching, frequent emesis, pain/irritation after meals, apneic episodes, recurrent respiratory infections); yet dysphagia-specific related symptoms were not specifically addressed in these guidelines.[56] There is literature support for reflux management improving dysphagia symptoms and signs in infants treated with 3 months of PPI therapy.[57] Their safety profile is considered generally favorable which supports use in infants; however, there are reports of increased rates of multisystem infection while using these medications which should be weighed when counseling patients and parents.[56,58,59]

CLINICS CARE POINTS

- Pediatric dysphagia is a common condition in high risk populations.
- Recognition and management of dysphagia is important to avoid respiratory and developmental sequelae.
- A multidisciplinary care team is vital in optimizing identification and management of pediatric dysphagia.

DISCLOSURE

The authors do not have any financial conflicts of interest to disclose related to this study.

REFERENCES

1. Ortiz Perez P, Valero Arredondo I, Torcuato Rubio E, et al. Clinicopathological characterization of children with dysphagia, family impact and health-related quality of life of their caregivers. An Pediatr 2022;96(5):431–40.
2. Casas MJ, McPherson KA, Kenny DJ. Durational aspects of oral swallow in neurologically normal children and children with cerebral palsy: an ultrasound investigation. Dysphagia 1995;10(3):155–9.
3. Mills N, Lydon AM, Davies-Payne D, et al. Imaging the breastfeeding swallow: Pilot study utilizing real-time MRI. Laryngoscope Investig Otolaryngol 2020;5(3):572–9.
4. Weckmueller J, Easterling C, Arvedson J. Preliminary temporal measurement analysis of normal oropharyngeal swallowing in infants and young children. Dysphagia 2011;26(2):135–43.
5. Cola PC, Afonso D, Baldelin CGR, et al. Oral transit time in children with neurological impairment indicated for gastrostomy. Codas 2020;32(2):e20180248.
6. Sasegbon A, Hamdy S. The anatomy and physiology of normal and abnormal swallowing in oropharyngeal dysphagia. Neuro Gastroenterol Motil 2017;29(11).
7. Steer KE, Johnson ML, Edmonds CE, et al. The Impact of Varying Nipple Properties on Infant Feeding Physiology and Performance Throughout Ontogeny in a

Validated Animal Model. Dysphagia 2023. https://doi.org/10.1007/s00455-023-10630-w.

8. Crary MA, Carnaby GD, Mathijs L, et al. Spontaneous Swallowing Frequency, Dysphagia, and Drooling in Children With Cerebral Palsy. Arch Phys Med Rehabil 2022;103(3):451–8.

9. Lau C, Smith EO. A novel approach to assess oral feeding skills of preterm infants. Neonatology 2011;100(1):64–70.

10. Koenig JS, Davies AM, Thach BT. Coordination of breathing, sucking, and swallowing during bottle feedings in human infants. J Appl Physiol 1990;69(5):1623–9.

11. Broussard DL, Altschuler SM. Central integration of swallow and airway-protective reflexes. Am J Med 2000;108(Suppl 4a):62S–7S.

12. Miller JL, Kang SM. Preliminary ultrasound observation of lingual movement patterns during nutritive versus non-nutritive sucking in a premature infant. Dysphagia 2007;22(2):150–60.

13. Goldfield EC, Buonomo C, Fletcher K, et al. Premature infant swallowing: patterns of tongue-soft palate coordination based upon videofluoroscopy. Infant Behav Dev 2010;33(2):209–18.

14. Rommel N, van Wijk M, Boets B, et al. Development of pharyngo-esophageal physiology during swallowing in the preterm infant. Neuro Gastroenterol Motil 2011;23(10):e401–8.

15. Ostadi M, Jokar F, Armanian AM, et al. The effects of swallowing exercise and non-nutritive sucking exercise on oral feeding readiness in preterm infants: A randomized controlled trial. Int J Pediatr Otorhinolaryngol 2021;142:110602.

16. Delaney AL, Arvedson JC. Development of swallowing and feeding: prenatal through first year of life. Dev Disabil Res Rev 2008;14(2):105–17.

17. Redstone F, West JF. The importance of postural control for feeding. Pediatr Nurs 2004;30(2):97–100.

18. Le Reverend BJ, Edelson LR, Loret C. Anatomical, functional, physiological and behavioural aspects of the development of mastication in early childhood. Br J Nutr 2014;111(3):403–14.

19. Committee on Injury, V. and P. Poison. Prevention of choking among children. Pediatrics 2010;125(3):601–7.

20. Peterson Lu E, Bowen J, Foglia M, et al. Etiologies of Poor Weight Gain and Ultimate Diagnosis in Children Admitted for Growth Faltering. Hosp Pediatr 2023;13(5):394–402.

21. Lefton-Greif MA, Okelo SO, Wright JM, et al. Impact of children's feeding/swallowing problems: validation of a new caregiver instrument. Dysphagia 2014;29(6):671–7.

22. Peetsold MG, Heij HA, Deurloo JA, et al. Health-related quality of life and its determinants in children and adolescents born with oesophageal atresia. Acta Paediatr 2010;99(3):411–7.

23. Thottam PJ, Simons JP, Choi S, et al. Clinical relevance of quality of life in laryngomalacia. Laryngoscope 2016;126(5):1232–5.

24. Smith CH, Jebson EM, Hanson B. Thickened fluids: investigation of users' experiences and perceptions. Clin Nutr 2014;33(1):171–4.

25. Okada J, Wilson E, Wong J, et al. Financial impacts and community resources utilization of children with feeding difficulties. BMC Pediatr 2022;22(1):508.

26. Tanaka N, Nohara K, Ueda A, et al. Effect of aspiration on the lungs in children: a comparison using chest computed tomography findings. BMC Pediatr 2019;19(1):162.

27. Gurberg J, Birnbaum R, Daniel SJ. Laryngeal penetration on videofluoroscopic swallowing study is associated with increased pneumonia in children. Int J Pediatr Otorhinolaryngol 2015;79(11):1827–30.

28. Pavithran J, Puthiyottil IV, Narayan M, et al. Observations from a pediatric dysphagia clinic: Characteristics of children at risk of aspiration pneumonia. Laryngoscope 2019;129(11):2614–8.

29. Speyer R, Cordier R, Kim JH, et al. Prevalence of drooling, swallowing, and feeding problems in cerebral palsy across the lifespan: a systematic review and meta-analyses. Dev Med Child Neurol 2019;61(11):1249–58.

30. Tanaka N, Nohara K, Uota C, et al. Relationship between daily swallowing frequency and pneumonia in patients with severe cerebral palsy. BMC Pediatr 2022;22(1):485.

31. Skinner ML, Lee SK, Collaco JM, et al. Financial and Health Impacts of Multidisciplinary Aerodigestive Care. Otolaryngol Head Neck Surg 2016;154(6):1064–7.

32. Bhattacharyya N. The prevalence of pediatric voice and swallowing problems in the United States. Laryngoscope 2015;125(3):746–50.

33. Available at: https://iddsi.org/About-Us/History#: ~ :text=Dysphagia%20(swallowing%20disorder)%20is%20broadly,protecting%20the%20airway%20from%20choking. Accessed November 21, 2023.

34. Black LI, Vahratian A and Hoffman HJ. Communication disorders and use of intervention services among children aged 3–17 years: United States, 2012 [NCHS Data Brief No. 205]. National Center for Health Statistics, Available at: https://www.cdc.gov/nchs/products/databriefs/db205.htm, 2015. Accessed November 21, 2023.

35. Benfer KA, Weir KA, Bell KL, et al. Oropharyngeal dysphagia and cerebral palsy. Pediatrics 2017;140(6):e20170731. https://doi.org/10.1542/peds.2017-0731.

36. Calis EAC, Veuglers R, Sheppard JJ, et al. Dysphagia in children with severe generalized cerebral palsy and intellectual disability. Dev Med Child Neurol 2008;50(8):625–30.

37. Jaffal H, Isaac A, Johannsen W, et al. The prevalence of swallowing dysfunction in children with laryngomalacia: A systematic review. Int J Pediatr Otorhinolaryngol 2020;139:110464. https://doi.org/10.1016/j.ijporl.2020.110464.

38. Newman LA, Keckley C, Petersen MC, et al. Swallowing function and medical diagnoses in infants suspected of dysphagia. Pediatrics 2001;108(6):e106. https://doi.org/10.1542/peds.108.6.e106.

39. Lefton-Greif MA, Arvedson JC. Pediatric feeding and swallowing disorders: state of health, population trends, and application of the international classification of functioning, disability, and health. Semin Speech Lang 2007;28:161–5.

40. Miller CK. Updates on pediatric feeding and swallowing problems. Curr Opin Otolaryngol Head Neck Surg 2009;17:194–9.

41. Gasparin M, Schweiger C, Manica D, et al. Accuracy of clinical swallowing evaluation for diagnosis of dysphagia in children with laryngomalacia or glossoptosis. Pediatr Pulmonol 2017;52(1):41–7.

42. Saad M, Afsah O, Baz H, et al. Clinical and videofluoroscopic evaluation of feeding and swallowing in infants with oropharyngeal dysphagia. Int J Pediatr Otorhinolaryngol 2021;150:110900.

43. Calvo I, Conway A, Henriques F, et al. Diagnostic accuracy of the clinical feeding evaluation in detecting aspiration in children: a systematic review. Dev Med Child Neurol 2016;58(6):541–53.

44. Jiang Jiin-Ling, Fu Shu-Ying, Wang Wan-Hsiang, et al. Validity and reliability of swallowing screening tools used by nurses for dysphagia: A systematic review. Tzu Chi Med J 2016;28(Issue 2):41–8.

45. Baqays A, Rashid M, Johannsen W, et al. What are parents' perceptions related to barriers in diagnosing swallowing dysfunction in children? A grounded theory approach. BMJ Open 2021;11(3):e041591.

46. Dodrill P, Gosa MM. Pediatric Dysphagia: Physiology, Assessment, and Management. Ann Nutr Metab 2015;66(Suppl 5):24–31.

47. Lefton-Greif MA. Pediatric dysphagia. Phys Med Rehabil Clin N Am 2008;19(4): 837–51.

48. Speyer R, Cordier R, Kim J-H, et al. Prevalence of drooling, swallowing, and feeding problems in cerebral palsy across the lifespan: A systematic review and meta-analyses. Dev Med Child Neurol 2019;61(11):1249–58.

49. van den Engel-Hoek L, Erasmus CE, van Hulst KC, et al. Children with central and peripheral neurologic disorders have distinguishable patterns of dysphagia on videofluoroscopic swallow study. J Child Neurol 2014;29(5):646–53.

50. Norman V, Zühlke L, Murray K, et al. Prevalence of Feeding and Swallowing Disorders in Congenital Heart Disease: A Scoping Review. Frontiers in Pediatrics 2022;10:843023.

51. Fishbein M, Branham C, Fraker C, et al. The incidence of oropharyngeal dysphagia in infants with GERD-like symptoms. JPEN J Parenter Enteral Nutr 2013;37(5):667–73.

52. American Speech-Language-Hearing Association (n.d), Pediatric Feeding and Swallowing. (Practice Portal). Retrieved November 28th, 2023, Available at: www. asha.org/practice-portal/clinical-topics/pediatric-dysphagia/. Accessed November 21, 2023.

53. Dusick A. Investigation and management of dysphagia. Semin Pediatr Neurol 2003;10(4):255–64.

54. Steele CM, Alsanei WA, Ayanikalath S, et al. The influence of food texture and liquid consistency modification on swallowing physiology and function: a systematic review. Dysphagia 2015;30(1):2–26. Erratum in: Dysphagia. 2015 Apr;30(2): 272-3. PMID: 25343878; PMCID: PMC4342510.

55. Gosa MM, Suiter DM, Kahane JC. Videofluoroscopic analysis to determine the effects of thickened liquids on oropharyngeal swallowing function in infants with respiratory compromise. 2022. Dysphagia Volume 19.

56. Duncan DR, Larson K, Rosen RL. Clinical Aspects of Thickeners for Pediatric Gastroesophageal Reflux and Oropharyngeal Dysphagia. Curr Gastroenterol Rep 2019;21(7):30.

57. Rosen R, Vandenplas Y, Singendonk M, et al. Pediatric Gastroesophageal Reflux Clinical Practice Guidelines: Joint Recommendations of the North American Society for Pediatric Gastroenterology, Hepatology, and Nutrition and the European Society for Pediatric Gastroenterology, Hepatology, and Nutrition. J Pediatr Gastroenterol Nutr 2018;66(3):516–54.

58. Suskind DL, Thompson DM, Gulati M, et al. Improved infant swallowing after gastroesophageal reflux disease treatment: a function of improved laryngeal sensation? Laryngoscope 2006;116(8):1397–403.

59. Lassalle M, Zureik M, Dray-Spira R. Proton Pump Inhibitor Use and Risk of Serious Infections in Young Children. JAMA Pediatr 2023;177(10):1028–38. https://doi.org/10.1001/jamapediatrics.2023.2900.

Oral and Pharyngeal Dysphagia in Adults

Karuna Dewan, MD

KEYWORDS

- Oropharyngeal dysphagia • Oral phase • Pharyngeal phase • Dysphagia • Bolus
- Mastication • Cricopharyngeal achalasia

KEY POINTS

- Oral and pharyngeal dysphagia are "transport" dysphagias involving impaired bolus preparation and/or transport through the pharynx to the esophagus.
- Oral phase dysphagia involves poor bolus preparation and timing.
- Pharyngeal phase dysphagia involves the disordered transportation through the upper esophageal sphincter often resulting in copious pharyngeal residue. This places patients at risk for aspiration.
- The workhorse methods of evaluation include the oral mechanisms examination, flexible endoscopic evaluation of swallowing and modified barium swallow.
- Oral and pharyngeal dysphagia are best managed with a combination of surgical and therapeutic interventions as well as control of the underlying systemic disease. Multidisciplinary management of dysphagia produces the best outcomes.

INTRODUCTION

Dysphagia is a symptom or a collection of symptoms of underlying anatomic abnormalities, or impairments and disorders in cognitive, sensory, and motor acts involved in the transport of, mainly, food and drink from the oral cavity toward the stomach. Oropharyngeal dysphagia refers to abnormalities affecting the upper esophageal sphincter (UES), pharynx, larynx, and/or tongue. The prevalence of oropharyngeal dysphagia in the general population has been estimated to range between 2.3% and 16%.[1] However, in patient populations pooled prevalence has been reported to be as high as 42% in stroke, 50.9% in cerebral palsy, and 72.4% in dementia.[2–4] Prevalence numbers may depend on the severity of underlying disease, screening or assessment tools used to identify dysphagia, and health care settings.[5] Elderly patients are the population most associated with oropharyngeal dysphagia. Dysphagia is by definition a symptom, which is the end result of a number of pathologies. Other

Department of Otolaryngology–Head and Neck Surgery, Louisiana State University Health – Shreveport, 501 Kings Highway, Shreveport, LA 71103, USA
E-mail address: Karuna.dewan@lsuhs.edu

Otolaryngol Clin N Am 57 (2024) 541–550
https://doi.org/10.1016/j.otc.2024.03.004
0030-6665/24/© 2024 Elsevier Inc. All rights reserved.

studies in this issue will address the specific etiologies of dysphagia including neurologic and cancer-related dysphagia. There are many causes of oropharyngeal dysphagia, including neuromuscular, drug-induced, and structural etiologies.

Dysphagia may lead to reduced efficiency and safety of swallowing, pulmonary complications, and reduced quality of life.[6] Patients with oropharyngeal dysphagia have difficulty transferring food from the mouth into the pharynx and esophagus to initiate the involuntary swallowing process. This may be accompanied by nasopharyngeal regurgitation, aspiration, and a sensation of residual food remaining in the pharynx. Abnormalities affecting the UES, pharynx, larynx, or tongue, in isolation or combination, result in oropharyngeal dysphagia affecting either or both transit and airway protection.

NORMAL ORAL AND PHARYNGEAL PHASES

A normal swallow has 3 distinct phases: oral, pharyngeal, and esophageal. The oral phase can further be subdivided into oral preparatory and oral propulsive stages. Disorders of swallowing are often categorized according to the swallowing phase that is impacted. Impairments of the oral and pharyngeal phases are sometimes referred to as "transfer" dysphagias.

The oral stage of swallowing is often divided into 2 steps. In the oral preparatory phase, for liquids, the bolus is sealed into the oral cavity by the tongue anteriorly and the hard palate posteriorly. For solids, the bolus is processed via mastication and manipulation. During oral propulsion, the tongue elevates to move the bolus posteriorly into the oropharynx. This bolus is held in the oropharynx until the pharyngeal phase begins.[7]

The oropharyngeal phase starts with the retraction of the tongue base and the palatoglossal folds prevent the re-entry of the bolus to the oral cavity. The hypoglossal nerves and pharyngeal plexus are very important to this step. Nasopharyngeal regurgitation is prevented by the palatopharyngeus and musculus uvulae acting together with the pharyngeal plexus providing innervation. Suprahyoid muscles pull the larynx under the retracting tongue base. This is mediated by the mandibular division of the trigeminal nerve, which innervates the anterior belly of the digastric and mylohyoid muscles, the facial nerve innervating the posterior belly of the digastric and stylohyoid, and C1 through ansa hypoglossi innervating the geniohyoid and thyrohyoid muscles.[7] The larynx is also protected by the sphincteric closure of the aryepiglottic folds, ventricular bands, and the true vocal folds—all of which depend on innervation from the recurrent laryngeal nerves. Retroflection of the epiglottis also provides airway protection. Sensation is mediated by the internal branch of the superior laryngeal nerve.

Once the bolus enters the laryngopharynx, it is transferred to the esophagus. This is done by squeezing the thyropharyngeus and relaxing the cricopharyngeus. Cricopharyngeal relaxation is triggered by the stretch that occurs as a result of hyolaryngeal elevation.[8] The larynx closes during pharyngeal transit and respiration restarts with the expiratory phase. All of these mechanisms require a high level of coordination. This is mediated by the central pattern generator, a network of neurons in the brainstem.[9]

ABNORMALITIES OF THE ORAL PHASE

Oral phase dysphagia is a subtype of oropharyngeal dysphagia that impacts the mouth alone. Disorders affecting the oral preparatory and oral propulsive phases usually result from impaired control of the tongue, although dental problems and oral incompetence may also be involved.[10] Poor oral health, including poor dentition, and poorly fitting dentures are a known predictor of aspiration pneumonia in vulnerable populations such as the elderly and chronically ill and has been linked to systemic disease, morbidity, and mortality. When eating solid foods, patients may have difficulty chewing and initiating swallows. When drinking liquids, patients may find it difficult to contain the liquid in the oral cavity before they swallow. As a result, the bolus may be lost, spilling prematurely into the unprepared pharynx. This can lead to aspiration. The tongue and facial muscles play a central role in sucking, mastication, and swallowing.[11] They play multiple roles in breakdown of food and mixing it with saliva to form a bolus. The movement of the tongue is controlled by the hypoglossal nerve, and the facial muscles are controlled by the facial nerve. Any damage to them causes paralysis and renders the tongue and facial muscles incapable of functioning properly. Injury to the hypoglossal or facial nerve can occur because of infection, drug toxicity, tumor, compression, trauma, and iatrogenic or unknown causes.[12,13] Injury to the hypoglossal or facial nerves is among the most commonly observed cranial nerve injuries.[13] Oral phase dysphagia is very commonly the result of tongue weakness following a stroke.

Saliva plays a critical role in alimentary events, allowing food to be initially processed, formed into a bolus, and subsequently transported through the oral cavity. Patients with salivary gland hypofunction often present with dysphagic complaints. Patients subjectively reporting difficulty swallowing had significantly lower salivary flow rates than patients without dysphagia complaints.[14] Patients with documented salivary hypofunction display significantly increased duration of the oral phase of swallowing in several conditions.[15] Xerostomia contributes to oral phase dysphagia. Polypharmacy contributes to xerostomia. Patients taking greater than 12 medications were significantly more likely to experience xerostomia than those who were taking fewer medications.[16]

Facial nerve paralysis can lead to difficulties with oral competence as well as tongue weakness. Facial nerve paralysis arises from a wide range of diagnoses with etiologies including stroke, Bell's palsy, viral infection, accidental or surgical trauma, or tumor. Oral competence refers to the maintenance of lip closure with sufficient strength to prevent anterior spillage of saliva, food, and fluid. Patients with impaired oral competence are unable to retain the bolus anteriorly. They may also be unable to adequately prepare a bolus.

The movement of the tongue is an important contributor to the oral-stage of swallowing. It plays a crucial role in maintaining a cohesive bolus while manipulating the bolus during mastication and propelling the bolus out of the oral cavity through the larynx. For example, in stroke patients, dysfunctions including reduced tongue pressure and lingual discoordination limit the efficacy of the oral phase of the swallow.[17] Tongue pressure has been reported as a good predictor of oral phase dysphagia.[18] Unilateral tongue weakness, also a contributor to oral phase dysphagia, is mostly caused by unilateral hypoglossal nerve injury or weakness.

ABNORMALITIES OF THE PHARYNGEAL PHASE

Dysfunction of the pharyngeal phase of swallowing leads to impairment of food transport to the esophagus. Food is retained in the pharynx after a swallow. When there is obstruction of the pharynx by a stricture, web or tumor, weakness or incoordination of the pharyngeal muscles or poor opening of the UES, patients may retain excessive amounts of food in the pharynx and experience overflow aspiration after swallowing. If pharyngeal clearance is severely impaired, patients may be unable to ingest sufficient calories to maintain their weight and hydration. A pharyngeal diverticulum may also impair pharyngeal emptying by diverting the bolus from its normal course. In addition, weakness of the soft palate and pharynx may lead to the nasal regurgitation of food.

The velopharyngeal valve is an area in the pharynx that creates a physical barrier between the nasal and oral cavities. This value closes during the functions of blowing, whistling, vomiting, swallowing, and for certain sounds during speech.[19] Velopharyngeal dysfunction is a general term for abnormal velopalatal (VP) movement or closure. The term velopharyngeal insufficiency is typically used to describe velopharyngeal dysfunction due to abnormal structure. The term velopharyngeal incompetence usually describes a disorder cause by abnormal neurophysiology because of congenital or acquired brain injury.[19] There is normal structure, but poor movement or discoordination of the velopharyngeal structures. Velopalatal insufficiency (VPI) can lead to dysphagia and often nasal regurgitation of food or liquid. Additionally, in the patient with VPI, enough propulsive force may not be generated to open the UES adequately as the oral and nasal cavities cannot be sealed off from each other. This leads to bolus retention within the pharynx and ultimately may place the patient at risk for aspiration.[20]

The larynx plays an important role in swallowing by protecting the airway through reflexes. Therefore, paralysis of any part of the larynx can lead to severe life-threatening complications. Two branches of the vagus nerve—the superior laryngeal nerve (SLN) and the recurrent laryngeal nerve (RLN)—innervate the laryngeal muscles on each side. The SLN runs toward the larynx and is divided into internal and external branches. The internal or sensory branch pierces the thyrohyoid membrane and is distributed to the upper larynx. The external branch (motor) innervates the cricothyroid muscles. The RLN innervates all intrinsic muscles of the larynx, except for the cricothyroid muscles. Most vocal fold paralysis is caused by RLN paralysis.[21] When the RLN is injured but the SLN is intact, sensation in the larynx remains and the cricothyroid muscle is not paralyzed. However, isolated SLN injury can occur after surgery, such as thyroidectomy or anterior approach to the cervical spine.[22] SLN injury or decreased sensation to the laryngeal vestibule may lead to aspiration as the patient is unable to sense the presence of the bolus within the laryngeal vestibule or further down in the airway. Unilateral vagal nerve injury has been noted to cause chronic bronchial aspiration.[21,23]

Dysphagia secondary to unilateral vocal fold paralysis or paresis (UVFP) can result in glottic incompetence, inefficient laryngeal closure, inefficient thyropharyngeal contraction, reduced laryngeal sensation, and impaired function of the UES. UVFP resultant dysphagia is of the utmost importance of those patients who have undergone thoracic and mediastinal surgeries. The risk of dysphagia in UVFP is increased by the inability of the bolus to develop adequate speed or consistency and compromised UES opening.[24] With injury, the airway may not be adequately protected during swallowing as the glottis is not able to fully close.[24] Management options for UVFP-associated dysphagia are aimed at improving glottal closure through injection laryngoplasty and type I thyroplasty. Injection laryngoplasty within 4.5 days of onset of UVFP is associated with decreased incidence of aspiration pneumonia and shortened length of hospital stay.[25–27]

Elevation of the larynx is critical to swallowing function. Impaired hyolaryngeal excursion and subsequent inadequate opening of the UES are commonly attributed to postradiation therapy dysphagia. Two muscle groups that suspend the hyoid, larynx, and pharynx have been proposed to elevate the hyolaryngeal complex: the suprahyoid and longitudinal pharyngeal muscles. The thyrohyoid is active in both groups. Elevation of the hyolaryngeal complex is central to the intricate set of movements required to transfer a bolus from the oral cavity through the hypopharynx and into the esophagus. The hyolaryngeal complex consists of the hyoid muscle, the laryngeal cartilages, and the muscles intrinsic to the hyoid and larynx, including the thyrohyoid. The cricopharyngeal muscle, the most inferior portion of the pharyngeal constrictor muscles, attaches to the hyolaryngeal complex and forms the UES.[28] Proper hyolaryngeal elevation draws the airway anterior to the trajectory of the oncoming bolus and stretches open a relaxed UES. Inadequate hyolaryngeal elevation can result in aspiration or bolus retention, putting the patient at risk of inadequate oral intake, need for an altered diet and pneumonia. Swallowing research argues that the suprahyoid and thyrohyoid muscles are primarily responsible for hyolaryngeal elevation and, therefore, the opening of the upper esophageal sphincter.[29]

Cricopharyngeal dysfunction refers broadly to the poor compliance of the UES or pharyngoesophageal segment resulting in reduced or absent opening during swallowing. It may result from primary neuromuscular dysfunction, mechanical obstruction, or stenosis of the UES, or discoordination of the UES opening with the rest of the swallow. The most common causes of cricpharyngeal muscle (CP) dysfunction are neurological disorders and the consequences, directly or indirectly, of head and neck cancer. Aging results in reduced CP compliance, strength, and muscle mass. Oral, pharyngeal, and esophageal dysfunctions also affect UES function. Depending on the severity of the dysfunction, symptoms may be absent or patients may complain of dysphagia, regurgitation, cough, aspiration, weight loss, dysphonia, and/or globus. Misdirection of the food bolus or penetration of the laryngeal vestibule may lead to cough, choking, and/or aspiration.[30,31] Bolus transit through the UES may be slowed by restricted UES opening, reduced pharyngeal driving pressures, and impaired hyolaryngeal elevation.

PRESENTING SYMPTOMS OF ORAL AND PHARYNGEAL DYSPHAGIA

Symptoms vary in both characteristics and severity, depending on the underlying disease state or injury. The consequences of dysphagia include malnutrition and dehydration, aspiration pneumonia, compromised general health, chronic lung disease, choking, and even death. Adults with dysphagia may also experience disinterest, reduced enjoyment, embarrassment, and/or isolation related to eating or drinking. Dysphagia may increase caregiver costs and burden and may require significant lifestyle alterations for the patient and the patient's family. Symptoms range from unreported, or silent, aspiration to frequent throat clearing to difficulty swallowing food resulting in aspiration. Common presenting symptoms are inability to keep the bolus in the oral cavity, difficulty gathering the bolus at the back of the tongue, difficulty initiating the swallow. As the bolus is supposed to progress through the upper aerodigestive tract, patients will feel food sticking in the throat. They may experience nasal regurgitation, inability to propel the bolus into the pharynx. This can manifest as difficulty swallowing swallows, frequent repetitive swallows, and frequent throat clearing. Patients may note voice changes including a wet voice or hoarse voice after meals, hypernasal voice, and dysarthria. Cough may be noted before, during, or after swallowing. Most concerning are unintended weight loss and recurrent pneumonia.

Not all signs and symptoms are seen in all types of dysphagia, and the evidence supporting the predictive value of these signs and symptoms is mixed. For example, coughing and throat clearing may not be correlated with penetration of aspiration of a bolus but may be the result of gastroesophageal reflux, esophageal dysmotility, or common medications.[4,5,32] Drooling and poor oral management of secretions, nasal regurgitation of foods and liquid, extra time needed to chew, as well as ineffective chewing and inability to maintain lip closure can be symptoms of oral dysphagia. Food or liquid remaining in the oral cavity after swallowing, complaints of food sticking, pain with swallowing, change in voice quality during or after eating, coughing/throat clearing during or after eating/drinking are all signs of pharyngeal dysphagia. Recurrent pneumonia, weight loss, malnutrition, and dehydration can also be signs/symptoms indicating of oropharyngeal dysphagia. Silent aspiration may be present as the patient presents without overt signs or symptoms of dysphagia. It is important to consider the signs and symptoms of dysphagia in the context of data points including the etiology of dysphagia and the overall health of the patient.

WORKUP

The workup for dysphagia will be addressed in a later section in this volume. However, it is important to note the workhorse methods of dysphagia evaluation for the oral and pharyngeal phases are the oral mechanism examination, flexible endoscopic evaluation of swallowing (FEES) and modified barium swallow (MBSS).[33] MBSS and FEES yield the best diagnostic information and indicate which therapeutic modalities are most appropriate. These techniques can also be utilized to evaluate response after patient treatment.

TREATMENT OF ORAL AND PHARYNGEAL DYSPHAGIA

As oral and pharyngeal dysphagia are often symptoms or manifestations of systemic disease, treatment involves the management of the underlying condition especially in the case of metabolic and neurologic disease. This will be addressed in subsequent sections. However, in some cases, surgical intervention is appropriate.

In the setting of cricopharyngeal achalasia/dysfunction, surgical intervention is warranted. This is helpful when there are conditions that cause dysfunction of bolus outflow from the pharynx to the esophagus. Typically, surgical methods are geared toward reducing sphincter tone or mechanically enhancing UES opening through myotomy and/or dilation. The current methods are best classified as either endoscopic or open surgical procedures. Endoscopic procedures include the injection of botulinum toxin into the CP muscle, CP myotomy, and dilation. These may be done independently or in any combination. Dilation of the CP can be done using a balloon dilator or with rigid dilators. Open surgical management involves accessing and dividing the CP muscle via a lateral cervical incision.[34]

Treatment of UVFP, regardless of technique, focuses on reducing glottic insufficiency through various means such as injection augmentation, medialization thyroplasty, arytenoid addiction, and RLN reinnervation. In adults, injection augmentation and medialization thyroplasty are the most utilized and accepted approaches in treating UVFP. In a systemic review, Dhar and colleagues demonstrate that the treatment of adults with vocal fold medialization procedures of injection augmentation or medialization thyroplasty can improve swallowing outcomes.[35]

Most patients with oropharyngeal dysphagia require physical rehabilitation through swallow therapy and dietary alteration. Dietary alterations require the participation of both the patient and their family members to modify the way food is prepared and to omit those foods that present a challenge in terms of swallowing. Some patients require soft or pureed foods. Others may require manipulation of bolus size. Dietary changes should focus on alleviating the difficulties of dysphagia while allowing for adequate nutrition and maintaining the patient's quality of life with respect to eating.

Swallow therapy, conducted by a speech language pathologist, is designed to strengthen the muscles involved in swallowing and enhance the quality of the mechanism. Treatment of dysphagia includes active exercises and other strategies, including compensations designed to improve the safety of the swallow and efficiency of surgical procedures, medications, and dental prosthetic devices.[36] Treatment of dysphagia involves 2 parallel approaches. First, the use of compensatory measures to allow the patient to eat, at least, some foods orally without aspiration. Second, the introduction of exercises to build strength and coordination so that patients no longer need the compensations and can return to full oral intake.[18] The simplest of these techniques involves several dry swallows following the swallow of food to enhance pharyngeal closure and reduce pharyngeal residue. In the super supraglottic swallow, the patient takes a deep breath and bears down while swallowing, followed by a cough, to close the airway and reduce aspiration. During Mendelsohn's maneuver, the patient generates a sustained laryngeal and hyoid bone elevation following the swallow to prolong the upper esophageal sphincter opening and enhance emptying. The Shaker maneuver is a regimen of isotonic and isometric head raises from a supine position to strengthen the traction forces of the suprahyoid muscles. There are also a variety of postural techniques that can be utilized, including chin tuck, chin-up, and head rotation or tilting, to promote safe passage of the food bolus and reduce or eliminate aspiration.

A multidisciplinary team (MDT) can track the patient's worsening swallow function and prove a stimulus to help the patient achieve better comfort, thus helping monitor this functional degradation, which could assist the team in the general clinical prognosis.[37] Oral and pharyngeal adult dysphagia being a complex disorder with many etiologies, anatomic regions of dysfunction, and potential treatments is a prime disorder for multidisciplinary evaluation. The greatest value of the multidisciplinary approach lies in the opportunity for assessment and treatment planning for patients with complex conditions where multiple practitioners carry unique expertise and skills.[38] The exact composition of the MDT may be different at each institution. However, it ideally involves otolaryngology, speech language pathology, and nutrition. A team may also include geriatrician, gastroenterology, neurology, dentistry/oral surgery, and radiation oncology depending upon the specific patient population with dysphagia. The causes of dysphagia and consequences of dysphagia cross the traditional boundaries between professional disciplines and may require the input of multiple medical or therapeutic specialists. The mouth, throat, upper airway, larynx, trachea, esophagus, and stomach are all involved in feeding and swallowing. Individuals with complex issues are best managed by an MDT of specialists.[39] Current research has established the benefits delivered through an integrated MDT approach in patients with amyotrophic lateral sclerosis (ALS), head and neck cancer, Parkinson disease, stroke, and so forth resulting in improved patient outcomes and better survival rates. Delivery of MDT services is also noted to maximize results, increase efficiency in care delivery, reduce costs, shorten the duration of hospitalization, and improve overall patient outcomes.

SUMMARY

Patients with oral and pharyngeal dysphagia have difficulty forming a cohesive bolus and/or transferring food from the mouth into the pharynx and esophagus to initiate the involuntary swallowing process. This may be accompanied by nasopharyngeal regurgitation, aspiration, and a sensation of residual food remaining in the pharynx. Abnormalities affecting the upper esophageal sphincter, pharynx, larynx, or tongue, in isolation or combination, result in oropharyngeal dysphagia affecting either or both transit and airway protection. These issues can be addressed with a combination of management of the underlying systemic disease, with surgical intervention or with swallow therapy. Dysphagia is a complex condition that is best served by multidisciplinary care.

CLINICS CARE POINTS

- Oral and pharyngeal dysphagia in the adult involves a malfunction of the ability to transport food/liquid through the pharynx to the esophageal inlet. This often presents coughing with oral intake, weight loss, and aspiration.
- Poor bolus preparation, the primary cause or oral phase dysphagia, can be caused by dentition problems, weakness of the tongue, and poor palatal motion.
- Pharyngeal phase dysphagia involves the disordered transportation through the upper esophageal sphincter often resulting in copious pharyngeal residue. This places patients at risk for aspiration.
- The MBSS and the flexible endoscopic evaluation of swallowing (FEES) are the primary instrumental tools to assess oral and pharyngeal dysphagia.
- Oral and pharyngeal dysphagia are best managed with a combination of surgical and therapeutic interventions as well as control of the underlying systemic disease.
- Multidisciplinary management of dysphagia produces the best outcomes.

DISCLOSURE

The above-listed authors do not have any commercial or financial conflicts of interest.

REFERENCES

1. Kertscher B, Speyer R, Fong E, et al. Prevalence of oropharyngeal dysphagia in the Netherlands: a telephone survey. Dysphagia 2015;30(2):114–20.
2. Banda KJ, Chu H, Chen R, et al. Prevalence of oropharyngeal dysphagia and risk of pneumonia, malnutrition, and mortality in adults aged 60 years and older: a meta-analysis. Gerontology 2022;68(8):841–53.
3. Rajati F, Ahmadi N, Naghibzadeh ZA, et al. The global prevalence of oropharyngeal dysphagia in different populations: a systematic review and meta-analysis. J Transl Med 2022;20(1):175.
4. Speyer R, Balaguer M, Cugy E, et al. Expert consensus on clinical decision making in the disease trajectory of oropharyngeal dysphagia in adults: an international delphi study. J Clin Med 2023;12(20).
5. Agnes CS, Nayak S, Devadas U. Prevalence of oropharyngeal dysphagia symptoms in community-dwelling older adults: A community survey. Indian J Gastroenterol 2023. https://doi.org/10.1007/s12664-023-01476-z.
6. Speyer R, Cordier R, Kertscher B, et al. Psychometric properties of questionnaires on functional health status in oropharyngeal dysphagia: a systematic literature review. BioMed Res Int 2014;2014:458678.
7. Matsuo K, Palmer JB. Anatomy and physiology of feeding and swallowing: normal and abnormal. Phys Med Rehabil Clin N Am 2008;19(4):691–707, vii.
8. Pearson WG Jr, Langmore SE, Yu LB, et al. Structural analysis of muscles elevating the hyolaryngeal complex. Dysphagia 2012;27(4):445–51.
9. Teasell R, Foley N, Fisher J, et al. The incidence, management, and complications of dysphagia in patients with medullary strokes admitted to a rehabilitation unit. Dysphagia 2002;17(2):115–20.

10. Charters E, Coulson S. Oral competence following facial nerve paralysis: Functional and quality of life measures. Int J Speech Lang Pathol 2021;23(2):113–23.
11. Charters E, Low TH, Coulson S. Utility of an oral competence questionnaire for patients with facial nerve paralysis. J Plast Reconstr Aesthetic Surg 2023;77: 201–8.
12. Welby L, Ukatu CC, Thombs L, et al. A mouse model of dysphagia after facial nerve injury. Laryngoscope 2021;131(1):17–24.
13. Odebode TO, Ologe FE. Facial nerve palsy after head injury: Case incidence, causes, clinical profile and outcome. J Trauma 2006;61(2):388–91.
14. Fox PC, Busch KA, Baum BJ. Subjective reports of xerostomia and objective measures of salivary gland performance. J Am Dent Assoc 1987;115(4):581–4.
15. Fox PC, van der Ven PF, Sonies BC, et al. Xerostomia: evaluation of a symptom with increasing significance. J Am Dent Assoc 1985;110(4):519–25.
16. Marcott S, Dewan K, Kwan M, et al. Where dysphagia begins: polypharmacy and xerostomia. Fed Pract 2020;37(5):234–41.
17. Daniels SK, Brailey K, Foundas AL. Lingual discoordination and dysphagia following acute stroke: analyses of lesion localization. Dysphagia 1999;14(2): 85–92.
18. Logemann JA. Treatment of oral and pharyngeal dysphagia. Phys Med Rehabil Clin N Am 2008;19(4):803–16, ix.
19. Lynch CA, Rule DW, Klaben B, et al. Surgical treatment of acquired velopharyngeal insufficiency in adults with dysphagia and dysphonia. J Voice 2022. https://doi.org/10.1016/j.jvoice.2021.12.003.
20. Abdelmeguid A, Rojansky R, Berry GJ, et al. Dysphagia and dysphonia, a pairing of symptoms caused by an unusual pair of diseases: castleman's disease and myasthenia gravis. Ann Otol Rhinol Laryngol 2021;130(3):319–24.
21. Dewan K, Vahabzadeh-Hagh A, Soofer D, et al. Neuromuscular compensation mechanisms in vocal fold paralysis and paresis. Laryngoscope 2017;127(7): 1633–8.
22. Sheahan P, Murphy MS. Thyroid Tubercle of Zuckerkandl: importance in thyroid surgery. Laryngoscope 2011;121(11):2335–7.
23. Havas T, Lowinger D, Priestley J. Unilateral vocal fold paralysis: causes, options and outcomes. Aust N Z J Surg 1999;69(7):509–13.
24. Kim CM, Dewan K. Vocal fold paralysis and dysphagia. Curr Otorhinolaryngol Rep 2021;9:101–6.
25. Chen DW, Price MD, LeMaire SA, et al. Early versus late inpatient awake transcervical injection laryngoplasty after thoracic aortic repair. Laryngoscope 2018; 128(1):144–7.
26. Barnes JH, Orbelo DM, Armstrong MF, et al. Cardiothoracic patients with unilateral vocal fold paralysis: pneumonia rates following injection laryngoplasty. Ann Otol Rhinol Laryngol 2020;129(11):1129–34.
27. Reder L, Bertelsen C, Angajala V, et al. Hospitalized patients with new-onset vocal fold immobility warrant inpatient injection laryngoplasty. Laryngoscope 2021;131(1):115–20.
28. Pearson WG Jr, Hindson DF, Langmore SE, et al. Evaluating swallowing muscles essential for hyolaryngeal elevation by using muscle functional magnetic resonance imaging. Int J Radiat Oncol Biol Phys 2013;85(3):735–40.
29. Heijnen BJ, Speyer R, Kertscher B, et al. Dysphagia, speech, voice, and trismus following radiotherapy and/or chemotherapy in patients with head and neck carcinoma: review of the literature. BioMed Res Int 2016;2016:6086894.

30. Chhetri DK, Dewan K. Dysphagia evaluation and management in otolaryngology. St. Louis, MO: Elsevier; 2019.

31. Hughes CV, Baum BJ, Fox PC, et al. Oral-pharyngeal dysphagia: A common sequela of salivary gland dysfunction. Dysphagia 1987;1:173–7.

32. Rofes L, Arreola V, Almirall J, et al. Diagnosis and management of oropharyngeal dysphagia and its nutritional and respiratory complications in the elderly. Gastroenterol Res Pract 2011;2011.

33. Coyle JL, Davis LA, Easterling C, et al. Oropharyngeal dysphagia assessment and treatment efficacy: setting the record straight (response to Campbell-Taylor). J Am Med Dir Assoc 2009;10(1):62–6 [discussion 79-83].

34. Dewan K, Santa Maria C, Noel J. Cricopharyngeal achalasia: management and associated outcomes-a scoping review. Otolaryngol Head Neck Surg 2020; 163(6):1109–13.

35. Dhar SI, Ryan MA, Davis AC, et al. Does medialization improve swallowing function in patients with unilateral vocal fold paralysis? a systematic review. Dysphagia 2022;37(6):1769–76.

36. Logemann JA. Levels of evidence supporting dysphagia interventions: where are we going? Semin Speech Lang 2006;27(4):219–26.

37. Silva DNM, Vicente LCC, Gloria VLP, et al. Swallowing disorders and mortality in adults with advanced cancer outside the head and neck and upper gastrointestinal tract: a systematic review. BMC Palliat Care 2023;22(1):150.

38. Starmer HM, Dewan K, Kamal A, et al. Building an integrated multidisciplinary swallowing disorder clinic: considerations, challenges, and opportunities. Ann N Y Acad Sci 2020;1481(1):11–9.

39. Dewan K, Clarke JO, Kamal AN, et al. Patient reported outcomes and objective swallowing assessments in a multidisciplinary dysphagia clinic. Laryngoscope 2021;131(5):1088–94.

Oral Structural Dysphagia in Children

Rose P. Eapen, MD[a], Amelia F. Drake, MD[b],*, Allison Keane, MD[b]

KEYWORDS

- Oral dysphagia • Cleft lip and palate • Ankyloglossia

KEY POINTS

- Oral causes of dysphagia in children include problems with mobility of the tongue, which can be attributable to a short lingual frenum.
- Though surgical lysis of the short lingual frenum (frenectomy) is now performed frequently, it is important to be sure that this is indeed the cause of the dysphagia.
- Cleft palate causes dysphagia as the infant cannot create suction required in breast or bottle-feeding.
- Other congenital craniofacial conditions such as craniofacial microsomia or Pierre Robin sequence may be associated with dysphagia due to severe mandibular hypoplasia.

PEDIATRIC ORAL CAVITY EMBRYOLOGY AND ANATOMY
Anatomy

The oral cavity is the entry to the digestive system. It contains different anatomic structures, including the lips, tongue, palate, and dentition (if erupted). The tongue fills much of the space in the oral cavity. The hard and soft palate, including the uvula, forms the roof of the mouth. It is lined with stratified squamous epithelium known as oral mucosa. The floor of the oral cavity is supported by the mylohyoid muscles. Bilaterally, the submandibular and sublingual salivary glands produce saliva, which helps moisten and lubricate the oral cavity.

The oral cavity is critical in the initial point of entry for food and water. If teeth are present, they help grind food into small pieces for digestion. The tongue then helps develop a food bolus to be swallowed. The tongue also has papillae or taste buds which detect taste. The palate serves to divide the oral cavity from the nasal cavity and permits the independent functioning of breathing and food intake.

[a] Pediatric Otolaryngology, Miller Children's Hospital, 2711 North Sepulveda Boulevard, #520, Manhattan Beach, CA 90505, USA; [b] Department of Otolaryngology–Head and Neck Surgery, University of North Carolina, 170 Manning Drive CB 7070, Houpt Physicians Office Building Room G190A, Chapel Hill, NC 27599-7070, USA
* Corresponding author.
E-mail address: amelia_drake@unc.edu

Otolaryngol Clin N Am 57 (2024) 551–557
https://doi.org/10.1016/j.otc.2024.02.012
0030-6665/24/© 2024 Elsevier Inc. All rights reserved.

Embryology

The oral cavity forms from both endodermal and ectodermal structures.[1] The upper lip forms early in embryogenesis from the facial prominences which develop from neural crest cells, mesoderm, and ectoderm. Lingual swellings develop on either side of the first pharyngeal arch during the 5th week of embryologic development and become the anterior two-thirds of the tongue. The median sulcus divides them. The copula forms from the second pharyngeal arch and some of the third and fourth pharyngeal arches and becomes the posterior third of the tongue. The terminal sulcus divides the tongue between the anterior and posterior parts.

The palate forms between the sixth and twelfth week of embryologic development. The frontonasal prominences form the primary palate and include anterior upper jaw and philtrum. The paired maxillary prominences fuse to form the secondary palate. Palatal shelves elevate to form the roof of the oral cavity.[2]

The upper lip derives from anteriorly migrating neural crest cells, the lower lip forms from fusion of the mandibular processes. A facial cleft develops when the maxillary and lateral nasal prominences fail to fuse.[3,4]

Dental development is a complicated process that starts in the 8th week of intrauterine growth with development of enamel organs. Four stages of development have been described.[3] Though an infant does not normally erupt teeth until between 6 and 12 months of age, dental problems can be associated with pain, infection, and other causes of dysphagia.

Pediatric Dysphagia

Pediatric dysphagia can be prompted by abnormalities in several different anatomic sites within the oral cavity. These include the tongue, the lingual frenum, abnormalities of the craniofacial skeleton, dental disease, or neurologic problems coordinating the structures of the oral cavity to effectively move food within the oral cavity and hence feed effectively.

Abnormalities of the tongue itself can affect mobility. Congenital tumors such as hamartoma, lymphangiomas, or hemangiomas can occur. Macroglossia refers to an enlarged tongue and this can be caused by several conditions. Tongue ties, discussed further below, are perceived as a common cause of dysphagia and limitation of tongue mobility; lip and buccal ties have also been blamed for difficulty with feeding in many infants who have these anatomic variants.[5]

The roof of the oral cavity, the palate (made up of the hard palate and soft palate), can be a cause of dysphagia if a cleft of the palate is present. Though cleft lip can disrupt breast-feeding, as the lips encircle the nipple in normal conditions, the inability to have an effective suck is the main contributor to dysphagia when cleft palate is present. Treatment of this condition relies on modalities that allow the fluid bolus to enter the oral cavity without need for suction. Lactation experts can help in this process and have helped keep babies with clefts from becoming malnourished.

Craniofacial abnormalities that involve the mouth and the jaws, such as micrognathia, macrosomia, craniofacial microsomia and nasal obstruction are associated with dysphagia. In the case of jaw deformities, there are many associated abnormalities of the gums or dentition. Early involvement of multidisciplinary cleft and craniofacial teams helps to optimize the care of these patients.

Infants with neurologic conditions may experience feeding difficulty. Hypoxic-ischemic encephalopathy (HIE) is a complication due to birth asphyxia. Neonatal encephalopathy due to HIE may result in insufficient oral muscular control. These infants will present with difficulty latching and coordinating milk transfer.

DISCUSSION: ORAL CAVITY ANOMALIES AND CONTRIBUTIONS TO DYSPHAGIA
Ankyloglossia

The lead candidate for cause and subsequent intervention of oral lesions causing dysphagia, if recent research and clinical referrals are to be believed, is ankyloglossia or tongue-tie, especially in an infant. The diagnosis of this problem and the number of frenotomies performed has increased at least 10 fold over the past 20 years[6] (**Fig. 1**).

Intervention can include reassurance, stretching exercises, laser excision in a dental office or lysis of the tongue tie in the office or operating room, depending on age of the patient, anatomy, and tolerance. Though considered mostly safe, a recent article described 47 major complications in 34 patients, likely an underappreciated and underreported problem.[7,]

Normally or when the procedure is successful, the patient, usually an infant, starts latching at the breast and feeding much more effectively without additional intervention. In some anecdotal cases, however, revision procedures are recommended and/or performed, which points to the challenge of either accurate diagnosis or effective treatment of this relatively simple condition in a single setting.

Described as a "niche industry", and largely promoted by dentists and lactation consultants, the enormous increase in numbers of the largely nonreimbursed procedure of tongue-tie release is causing alarm among pediatricians and many others who care for very young children. With little oversight, the laser in-office procedure has been widely advertised and employed by dental practices. It is hoped that this procedure, like others, can be subjected to more study, and scrutiny of its results, in the future.[8]

Lip Tie/Buccal Tie

Other concerns within the anterior oral cavity are either buccal or labial ties. These are diagnosed along with tongue tie on many occasions though they do not appear as much to prohibit effective movement of oral structures.[9] The lip tie is thought to prevent the upper lip from surrounding the nipple of the breast to effectively nurse. Studies evaluating the importance of the lip tie to feeding, maxillary growth and future facial development are limited. The correction of lip ties is straight-forward but

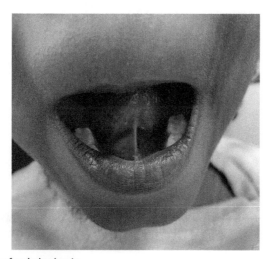

Fig. 1. Condition of ankyloglossia.

sometimes (anecdotally) associated with more of a "grimace" appearance to the smile than occurred previously. Buccal ties are lateral ties of the cheek, preventing mobilization of the food or milk bolus. Treatment of these can be controversial and has not been well studied. Surgery is not recommended in most cases though physical therapy or the recommended stretching exercises can be challenging to perform.

Macroglossia

Abnormalities of the tongue can be associated with significant dysphagia as well. Macroglossia, hemangiomas, or other congenital lesions can all affect mobility and effectiveness of tongue mobility. These can be varied in their severity or cause. Treatment would be adjusted to the cause and concomitant symptoms associated with the macroglossia.

Some congenital conditions associated with macroglossia include Trisomy 21, Beckwith Wiedemann, and the mucopolysaccharidoses. In the first two of these examples, the macroglossia can be evident early on. The facial features associated with mucopolysaccharidoses, including relative macroglossia, become, in contrast, more obvious over time (**Fig. 2**).

Cleft Lip and Palate

The presence of cleft lip and/or palate is frequently associated with difficulty feeding in the affected newborn infant. Whereas lip competence is needed to help the baby feed at the breast, a cleft of the palate makes the needed suction of the food or fluid impossible. Though many times clefts of the lip can be diagnosed at the time of a prenatal diagnostic ultrasound, cleft palate can be more challenging to visualize prenatally. Examination of the oral cavity is considered part of the newborn examination, but, surprisingly, some clefts of the soft palate are not noted for months after this time. The newborn examination also includes evaluation of the ears, and sometimes the finding of low-set or abnormal external ears promotes further work-up for a genetic condition.

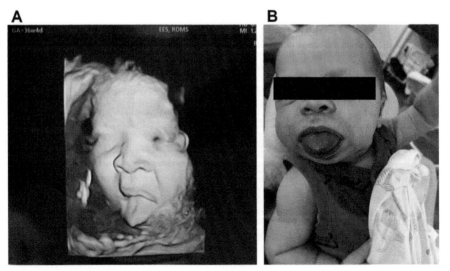

Fig. 2. Macroglossia diagnosed in utero by ultrasound, and in the same baby ex utero (*A, B*).

Around the world, cleft lip and palate patients are noted to have significant and at times life-threatening nutritional challenges. Their surgical success can depend on adequate nutritional status.[10]

Submucous cleft palate is a variant of cleft palate with a variable degree of velopharyngeal dysfunction resulting in dysphagia. Presentation can include bifid uvula, translucent zone in the soft palate, and notch in the posterior bony aspect of the hard palate[11,12] (**Fig. 3**).

Craniofacial Causes

The authors have noted the presence of swallowing dysfunction in patients with craniofacial conditions with marked mandibular hypoplasia, such as craniofacial microsomia.[13] Dysphagia, as well as airway symptoms, can be an early predictor of the need for medical intervention. The most important issue is the timely diagnosis and referral of such congenital conditions to multidisciplinary centers that include feeding teams. Adjuncts to oral feeding are required in some cases, to effectively nourish a child with a craniofacial condition, if it is severe. Also, it may be difficult to assess the contribution of the mandibular hypoplasia to the challenges with feeding noted with infants with Pierre Robin Sequence or Stickler's syndrome, as a cleft of the palate may coexist.

Nasal Obstruction

Congenital nasal obstruction is an important cause of neonatal dysphagia as infants are obligate nasal breathers during the first 3 months of life. Causes of nasal obstruction in the neonatal period vary in severity and include idiopathic (neonatal rhinitis), craniofacial (pyriform aperture stenosis, choanal atresia), and masses (dacryocystocele, teratoma, hairy polyp).[14] Management can vary depending on disease process. Some children will require an alternate feeding method until the primary cause of their nasal obstruction is adequately managed.[15]

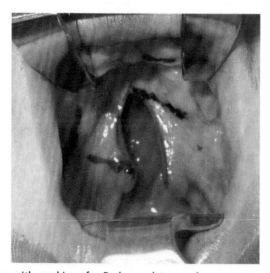

Fig. 3. Cleft palate, with markings for Furlow palate repair.

Dental Abnormalities

Salivary gland function or dental abnormalities can involve dysphagia as well. These can be related to congenital conditions such as ectodermal dysplasia or be secondary problems resulting from gastroesophageal reflux. As the dentition is an important element of the chewing of food and ability to make it of a consistency to effectively swallow, the importance of recognizing dental and gum disease is paramount in patients with feeding problems.

SUMMARY

As the oral cavity is the entry point of food or liquids entering a child for the purpose of nourishment, it is the initial site of evaluation for problems with such. Tongue tie is frequently listed as the culprit, with or without a comprehensive examination. Treatment of such, though frequently benign, can also cause pain, bleeding, or airway compromise and should not be considered unless truly indicated. Cleft lip and/or palate should be diagnosed, if present, in patients with poor feeding. Alternate nutritional support may be needed prior to or after surgical repair, that is, gastric feeding tube. Abnormalities of the jaws can cause limitation in oral intake, such as in infants with retrognathia. These are addressed over time, depending on the degree and anatomy involved. Lastly, dental or salivary gland disease can cause limitation in oral intake. In these instances, treatment is directed toward the pathology that is noted.

CLINICS CARE POINTS

- Oral causes of dysphagia can relate to abnormalities of the lips, tongue, the jaws, the palate, or the teeth.
- A common referral from lactation consultants relates to the presence of ankyloglossia.
- Addressing ankyloglossia surgically, usually safe, can have unexpected complications such as pain, bleeding, or airway compromise and should only be done if indicated.
- The presence of cleft lip and palate should be recognized early on and those patients referred to a multidisciplinary care team for optimal results.

DISCLOSURE

The authors have no financial disclosures.

REFERENCES

1. Netters Atlas of Human Anatomy, 6th edition, Frank H. Netter, MD. Epub.
2. Rinkoff S, Adlard RE. Embryology, craniofacial growth, and development. Available at: https://www.ncbi.nlm.nih.gov/books/NBK572156/.
3. Kamrani P, Nazia M. Anatomy, head and neck, oral cavity (mouth). Treasure Island (FL): StatPearls Publishing; 2023.
4. Jheon AH, Seidel K, Biehs B, et al. From molecules to mastication: the development and evolution of teeth. Wiley Interdiscip Rev Dev Biol 2013;2(2):165–82 [PMC free article] [PubMed].
5. Solis-Pazmin P, Kim GS, Lincango-Naranjo E, et al. Major complications after tongue-tie release: a case report and systematic review. Int J Pediatr Otorhinolaryngol 2020;138:110356.

6. Messner AH, Walsh J, Rosenfeld RM, et al. Clinical consensus statement: anky-loglossia in children. Otolaryngol Head Neck Surg 2020;162(5):597–611.

7. Dixon B, Gray J, Elliot N, et al. A multifaceted programme to reduce the rate of tongue-tie release surgery in newborn infants: observational study. J Pediatr Oto-rhinolaryngol 2018;113:156–63.

8. Available at: https://www.nytimes.com/2023/12/18/health/tongue-tie-release-breastfeeding.html.

9. Santa Maria C, Aby J, Truong MT, et al. The superior labial frenulum in newborns: what is normal? Glob Pediatr Health 2017;4. 2333794X17718896.

10. Delage B, Stieber E, Sheeran P. Prevalence of malnutrition among children at pri-mary cleft surgery: A cross-sectional analysis of a global database. J Glob Health 2022;12:04012.

11. Swibel Rosenthal LH, Walsh K, Thompson DM. Velopharyngeal incompetence: role in paediatric swallowing deficits. Curr Opin Otolaryngol Head Neck Surg 2018;26(6):356–66.

12. Dam E, van der Heijden P, Korsten-Meijer AG, et al. Age of diagnosis and eval-uation of consequences of submucous cleft palate. Int J Pediatr Otorhinolaryngol 2013;77(6):1019–24.

13. van de Lande LS, Cornelia JJMC, Pluijmers BI, et al. Evaluation of swallow func-tion in patients with craniofacial microsomia: a retrospective study. Dysphagia 2018;33(2):234–42.

14. Thiago LI, Pfeilsticker L, Silva V, et al. Eulalia Sakano Newborn nasal obstruction due to congenital nasal pyriform aperture stenosis. Allergy Rhinol 2016;7(1): 37–41.

15. Andres A, Villarroel G, Sedano C. Neonatal nasal obstruction. Eur Arch Oto-Rhino-Laryngol 2021;278(10):3605–11.

Laryngeal Structural Dysphagia in Children

Allison Keane, MD, Lauren K. Leeper, MD, Amelia F. Drake, MD*

KEYWORDS

- Pediatric dysphagia • Laryngomalacia • Vocal cord paralysis • Laryngeal cleft
- Subglottic stenosis

KEY POINTS

- The embryologic development of the laryngotracheal structures and esophagus is closely intertwined, and disruption to this process affects the functionality of both.
- Laryngotracheal anomalies as well as their surgical treatments impact the swallow function of pediatric patients.
- Laryngomalacia is the most common cause of pediatric stridor and is often associated with feeding difficulties in infants due to disruption of the suck–swallow–breathe mechanism.
- Laryngotracheal anomalies that narrow the pediatric airway can exacerbate gastroesophageal reflux, which worsens laryngotracheal inflammation.
- Clinical swallow evaluations are critical in patients with laryngotracheal pathology to identify aspiration.

INTRODUCTION
Pediatric Laryngeal Embryology and Anatomy

Embryology

The esophagus and laryngotracheal structures arise from the primitive foregut. In weeks 3 and 4 of gestation, a tracheobronchial groove develops from the foregut. A tracheoesophageal septum arises from the foregut at the carina and extends cranially to divide the future larynx and trachea from the esophagus. By the 6th week, the septum extends to the first tracheal ring. The cricoid ring is complete by the 7th week of gestation. The laryngeal cartilage and musculature develop from the 4th and 6th branchial arches. Abnormalities or disruptions in the development of the laryngotracheal structures can lead to respiratory and swallowing dysfunction in an infant.

Department of Otolaryngology–Head and Neck Surgery, University of North Carolina, 170 Manning Drive CB 7070, Physicians Office Building Room G190A, Chapel Hill, NC 27599-7070, USA
* Corresponding author.
E-mail address: Amelia_Drake@unc.edu

Otolaryngol Clin N Am 57 (2024) 559–568
https://doi.org/10.1016/j.otc.2024.02.014
0030-6665/24/© 2024 Elsevier Inc. All rights reserved.

oto.theclinics.com

Anatomy

The anatomy of the pediatric larynx is different from that of an adult. The larynx continues to develop as one ages. The pediatric larynx is located at a higher level in the neck, often between the C3 and C4 vertebrae in a full-term infant, and sometimes higher is a preterm infant. The narrowest portion of the pediatric larynx is the cricoid cartilage. The angle and shape of the epiglottis and vocal cords differ in children. The epiglottis is more narrow and curled in pediatric patients compared to adults. Adult vocal cords are typically more perpendicular with the trachea; the anterior insertion of the pediatric vocal cords is more inferior than the posterior insertion.

The high position of the larynx functionally separates the respiratory and digestive tracts. The epiglottis extends superior to the soft palate edge. The epiglottis assists in diverting oral boluses away from the airway to prevent aspiration. The positioning also results in a pause in respiration during swallowing, and a normal infant swallow follows the suck–swallow–breathe sequence. The anatomy also explains why infants are obligate nasal breathers. As the patient grows and develops, the laryngeal structures descend, the pharynx elongates, and the neuromuscular control of the structures develops, including the laryngeal adductor reflex. Afferent input from the superior laryngeal nerve from material in the supraglottis or glottis signals glottic closure through the recurrent laryngeal nerves.

Pediatric dysphagia

During the pharyngeal phase of the pediatric swallow, the vocal cords close, the larynx elevates and opens the esophageal inlet, and the epiglottis retroflexes. Anatomic abnormalities of the larynx mostly affect the pharyngeal swallow phase. A normal infant swallow follows a suck–swallow–breathe sequence. Any anatomic abnormality, such as laryngotracheal anomalies, that interferes with this sequence will interfere with the normal swallow. Infants with baseline difficulty breathing may struggle with the suck–swallow–breathe sequence.

Instrumental assessment of the swallow includes videofluoroscopic swallow study (VFSS) or fiberoptic endoscopic evaluation (FEES). VFSS allows visualization of all phases of the swallow and the degree of aspiration. It also allows for the assessment of improvement in swallow with certain therapeutic maneuvers. However, it requires radiation exposure, and there are limitations on patient positioning during the swallow. FEES provides visualization of airway structure before and after swallow, can assess secretion management, and does not require radiation. FEES can also be used to evaluate breastfeeding in infants. While a FEES is minimally invasive, there are small risks associated, and visualization during an active swallow is limited. Penetration and aspiration are common findings on swallow evaluations for patients with laryngeal anomalies. Penetration is spillage of material through the arytenoids to the vocal cords. Aspiration is the passage of the material through the vocal cords. Aspiration can lead to respiratory failure, aspiration pneumonias, and chronic lung disease.

Discussion: Laryngeal Anomalies and Contributions to Dysphagia

Laryngomalacia

Laryngomalacia is the most common congenital laryngeal anomaly and most common cause of pediatric stridor. It typically presents with inspiratory stridor exacerbated by supine positioning, feeding, crying, and agitation. Feeding is often disrupted by the need for multiple breaks, and patients commonly exhibit signs and symptoms of reflux, such as back arching and regurgitation. Symptoms typically present in the first few weeks of life and worsen before improving. Most patients will be symptom free by 12 to 18 months of age.

Initial physical examination may be significant for stridor, nasal flaring, subcostal and substernal retractions, and low-weight percentile. Severe forms of laryngomalacia may present with pectus excavatum, cor pulmonale, cyanosis, and failure to thrive. Failure to thrive can result from laryngomalacia secondary to the energy expenditure from work of breathing and difficulty with feeding. Diagnosis is confirmed with flexible fiberoptic laryngoscopy. Common findings on laryngoscopy are anatomic and mechanical, including a curled, omega-shaped epiglottis, posterior displacement of the epiglottis, short aryepiglottic folds, and redundant, prolapsing arytenoids (**Fig. 1**). Ideally, an objective assessment of dysphagia in patients with laryngomalacia includes VFSS and FEES evaluations.

The association between laryngomalacia and feeding difficulty is complex. The increased work of breathing in laryngomalacia can disrupt the suck–swallow–breathe mechanism in infants, causing difficulty with feeding. Also presented as a cause for feeding difficulty in laryngomalacia is the disruption of the laryngeal adductor reflex.[1] The true prevalence of subjective and objective dysphagia is unknown. Clinical assessment of swallowing function should be performed in patients with symptoms and should be considered for all patients with laryngomalacia even in the absence of dysphagia symptoms. Simons and colleagues report signs and symptoms of dysphagia subjectively reported in about 50% of patients with laryngomalacia.[2] In their review, 80.8% of patients with laryngomalacia and reported dysphagia symptoms had an abnormal instrumental swallow assessment, and 66.2% of patients with laryngomalacia without subjective dysphagia also had an abnormal instrumental swallow assessment.[2] Irace and colleagues found that 35.9% of patients with laryngomalacia underwent modified barium swallow study to evaluate for feeding difficulties based on history of recurrent respiratory issues and/or feeding difficulties.[3] Of those patients, 28.2% had laryngeal penetration and 42.3% had aspiration (98.3% of which was silent aspiration).[3] They hypothesized that silent aspiration occurs in 14.9% to 41.5% of patients with laryngomalacia.[3] The association between laryngomalacia and dysphagia is further complicated by the contribution of additional comorbidities to both diagnoses such as neurologic disorders, genetic abnormalities, gastroesophageal reflux disease (GERD), prematurity, or other laryngeal or esophageal anomalies.

Laryngomalacia is frequently associated with GERD. Simons and colleagues report 69.8% of patients with laryngomalacia were diagnosed with GERD, and it was more common in patients with moderate-or-severe laryngomalacia.[2] Chronic acidic exposure can alter laryngeal sensation and the laryngeal adductor reflex. It can also cause edema of the supraglottic tissues and exacerbate prolapse of the arytenoid tissues. The increased intrathoracic pressure generated during inspiration by patients with a narrow airway can increase the reflux of gastric contents. Laryngomalacia

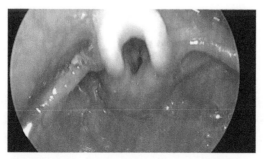

Fig. 1. Laryngomalacia with curled epiglottis and short aryepiglottic folds.

exacerbates GERD, which in turn exacerbates laryngomalacia. GERD may be primary or secondary to laryngomalacia.

Treatment of laryngomalacia is medical and/or surgical, depending on the severity. Medical treatment involves reflux management medications, positioning, and dysphagia therapy. Mild and moderate forms of laryngomalacia can often be managed without surgical intervention. Severe forms of laryngomalacia associated with failure to thrive, respiratory or cardiac complications require surgical intervention. About 10% of patients require surgical treatment. Surgery commonly addresses shortened aryepiglottic folds and redundant arytenoid or epiglottic tissue. Common techniques include cold dissection and laser ablation. Complications include stenosis secondary to scarring, and overaggressive resection can lead to worsened dysphagia and aspiration. Continued treatment of reflux is recommended to reduce the risk of complications.

Reports of dysphagia postsupraglottoplasty are varied. Ritcher and colleagues demonstrated improvement in laryngeal penetration and aspiration postoperatively from cold-knife supraglottoplasty.[1] Nguyen and colleagues found postoperative dysphagia on instrumental assessment in 65% of patients in the immediate postoperative period when only 42.5% had preoperative dysphagia.[4] Dysphagia should be assessed postoperatively in patients undergoing supraglottoplasty regardless of preoperative symptoms with special attention during the immediate postoperative period. Oral nutrition should be pursued only when clinically appropriate.

Laryngeal and subglottic stenosis

Subglottic stenosis is narrowing of the subglottic airway. Stenosis can be congenital or acquired. Congenital stenosis results from failure of recanalization of the larynx during development. Acquired stenosis is associated with trauma, intubation, inflammation, and reflux. Stenosis is graded based on the Cotton–Myer classification and the degree of airway narrowing.[5] Grade 1 stenosis is 50% or less obstruction. A 51% to 70% narrowed lumen is classified as grade 2 stenosis (**Fig. 2**A). Grade 3 stenosis is a 71% to 99% narrowed lumen, and grade 4 stenosis has no detectable lumen (**Fig. 2**B).

Laryngeal stenosis is narrowing of the glottic region of the airway. Laryngeal webs are a congenital malformation due to the failure of recanalization of the larynx (**Fig. 3**). While they can be an isolated occurrence, they are associated with 22q11 deletion and additional congenital malformations. Webs are classified according to the Cohen classification.[6] Type 1 webs are thin, narrowing the airway by less than 35%. Type 2 webs

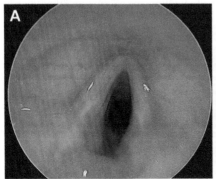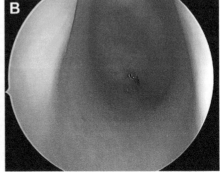

Fig. 2. (A) Grade 2 subglottic stenosis in comparison to (B) grade 4 subglottic stenosis.

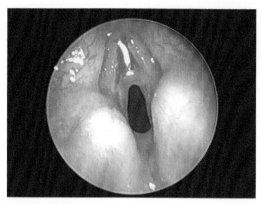

Fig. 3. Laryngeal web before endoscopic division.

narrow the airway by 35% to 50% and are moderately thick with associated subglottic stenosis. The airway is narrowed 50% to 75% with subglottic stenosis in type 3 webs. Type 4 webs narrow the airway between 75% and 95% again with significant subglottic stenosis.

Laryngeal and subglottic cysts are fluid-filled lesions in the mucosa. History of intubation or trauma to the larynx or subglottis is a risk factor for the development of a cyst. Presentation of a laryngeal or subglottic cyst resembles that of other causes of stenosis as the cyst similarly narrows the airway.

Laryngeal and subglottic stenosis present most commonly with respiratory symptoms that can range from recurrent croup or intermittent dyspnea to biphasic stridor and respiratory distress. Severity of symptoms commonly correlates with the degree of airway obstruction. Dysphagia may or may not be present in patients with airway obstruction and when present, may be multifactorial. Infants with severe airway obstruction can have difficulty with the suck–swallow–breathe sequence, resulting in dysphagia and even failure to tolerate oral nutrition. As discussed with laryngomalacia, airway obstruction increases intrathoracic pressure that can exacerbate GERD. Chronic acid exposure leads to chronic inflammation that exacerbates stenosis.

Treatment of laryngeal and subglottic stenosis can be categorized as endoscopic or open. Laryngeal cysts are amenable to lysis and may only require one intervention. Mild, thin laryngeal webs are amenable to endoscopic division with cold steel, laser, or ablation techniques. Soft subglottic stenosis can similarly be endoscopically divided, and balloon dilated. This is often accompanied by steroid injection to the affected area and serially repeated. More mature, cartilaginous stenosis can be addressed with endoscopic or open laryngotracheal reconstruction in which donor cartilage (costal, auricular, or laryngeal) is used to expand the airway. In severe grade 3 or grade 4 stenosis, cricotracheal resection can be performed to remove the stenotic segment. Tracheostomy is utilized to bypass severe airway obstruction as patients grow and are treated with various surgical interventions until a safe airway can be achieved.

Dysphagia following airway reconstructive procedures is varied. It ranges from mild to severe and can be transient or long-term. Surgery itself alters the laryngotracheal anatomy and widens the airway. As a result, protection of the airway during swallowing is altered which can increase aspiration. Compensatory mechanisms, swallowing exercises, diet modifications, and positioning modifications may combat this. Kou and colleagues demonstrated that patients undergoing posterior cartilage graft laryngotracheoplasty may have temporary postoperative swallowing dysfunction, but all patients tolerating oral nutrition preoperatively were able to return to their preoperative diet.[7] Postoperative dysphagia after laryngotracheal reconstruction is increased in the setting of concurrent procedures that additionally widen or affect supraglottic structures and the use of stents.[8] Patients with preoperative feeding difficulty are also more likely to have difficulty postoperatively.[8] Postoperative dysphagia is also complicated by comorbidities in patients undergoing surgery.

Vocal cord paralysis

Pediatric vocal cord paralysis can be unilateral or bilateral and congenital or iatrogenic. Congenital paralysis is more commonly bilateral, and iatrogenic paralysis is more commonly unilateral. Vocal cord paralysis is associated with cardiac, mediastinal, and neurologic anomalies that interfere with the vagus nerves or recurrent laryngeal nerves and/or the attempts to treat those anomalies that risks injury to the same. The vagus nerves exit the skull base at the jugular foramen and travel inferiorly in the neck along the carotid artery. The recurrent laryngeal nerves branch off in the mediastinum with the right recurrent laryngeal nerve looping under the right subclavian artery and traveling superiorly in the tracheoesophageal groove to the larynx. The left recurrent laryngeal nerve loops under the aortic arch and is closely associated with the ductus arteriosus prior to traveling superiorly in the left tracheoesophageal groove to the larynx. Compression, traction, or iatrogenic injury to either vagus nerve or recurrent laryngeal nerve along this course can lead to vocal cord paralysis. Birth trauma can cause traction on the nerves and subsequent paralysis as well. However, not all vocal cord paralysis is related to nerve injury. Arytenoid dislocation and cricoarytenoid fixation related to traumatic intubation or airway manipulation can result in vocal cord paralysis. Posterior glottis stenosis and scarring can limit vocal cord motion. In the absence of an identifiable etiology, vocal cord paralysis may be idiopathic.

Paralyzed vocal cords can limit airway patency, and patients may present with stridor or respiratory compromise. Less severe symptoms include dysphonia or a weak cry. Unilateral vocal cord paresis can have a similar although usually less severe respiratory presentation as bilateral vocal cord paresis. Patients with bilateral or unilateral vocal cord paralysis also commonly present with dysphagia and feeding difficulties. Due to vocal cord paralysis, during the pharyngeal phase of the pediatric swallow, the vocal cords may fail to close, which can lead to aspiration. Decreased laryngeal sensation and cough reflex in vocal cord paralysis can also increase the risk of aspiration.

Diagnosis can be made with flexible fiberoptic nasolaryngoscopy and visualization of the movement of the vocal cords. Patients developing symptoms postoperatively from a procedure involving the course of the recurrent laryngeal nerves require a flexible fiberoptic nasolaryngoscopy to confirm the diagnosis. Evaluation of a patient without a known etiology for vocal cord paralysis should include imaging of the head, neck, and chest that covers the course of the recurrent laryngeal nerve to assess for anomalies. Direct laryngoscopy and bronchoscopy under anesthesia allows for palpation of the cricoarytenoid joints and cords to assess passive mobility and is beneficial in circumstances in which intubation trauma, glottic stenosis, cricoarytenoid, or secondary airway anomalies are suspected.

Patients with vocal cord paralysis also require objective assessment of their swallow function with a VFSS and/or FEES. Assessment by speech and language pathologists for a safe swallow is critical because the dysphagia may not be overt. Irace and colleagues reported silent aspiration in 57% of patients with unilateral vocal cord paralysis.[9] Dysphagia associated with vocal cord paralysis is complex as it can be strictly related to the laryngeal etiology, or multifactorial and related to comorbidities or recent procedures irrespective of the vocal cord paralysis. Interventions with positioning, exercises, and different consistencies may be adequate. Enteral nutrition, temporarily or permanently, may be necessary in some cases as well.

Treatment of vocal cord paralysis depends on cause. Underlying cardiac, mediastinal, or neurologic causes may be treatable with secondary improvement to vocal cord paralysis, improving the airway and feeding symptoms. Iatrogenic injury secondary to a procedure may be temporary or permanent depending on the nature of the injury to the nerve, traction versus transection. Recovery of vocal cord mobility can also range from mild improvement to resolution and is expected to occur within 1 year from onset. Idiopathic paralysis can also resolve with time. Bilateral congenital idiopathic vocal cord paralysis is reported to spontaneously recover in 60% to 65% of patients.[10,11] However, dysphagia improvement has not been shown to correlate with vocal cord recovery in bilateral or unilateral vocal cord paralysis.[12,13] Unilateral or bilateral vocal cord paralysis requires close observation as the patient's airway symptoms and dysphagia will change with growth and development.

Management includes assessing if the patient has a safe airway and safe nutrition. A variety of surgical procedures can be utilized to address airway patency. In bilateral vocal cord paralysis, cordotomy, arytenoid lateralization, posterior cricoid grafting, and laryngotracheal reconstruction can be utilized to widen the airway. However, these may have permanent deleterious effects on the airway and voice. These may also worsen feeding difficulties and aspiration. Tracheostomy is a definitive airway that bypasses glottic obstruction from vocal cord paralysis.

Patients with an adequate airway in unilateral vocal cord paralysis mainly suffering from dysphagia and aspiration may benefit from injection laryngoplasty and medialization of the paralyzed vocal cord. Injection laryngoplasty involves injection of an absorbable material into the paralyzed vocal cord to minimize the glottic incompetence. Injection has been proven to allow initiation of an oral diet or advancement of a previously restricted diet in pediatric patients with vocal cord paralysis, and the procedure is associated with a low rate of complications.[14] Results were improved for those that underwent injection within 6 months of onset of paralysis.[14] The injection is temporary and therefore beneficial in patients undergoing observation for potential vocal cord recovery. Additionally, the procedure provides input into the expected response from a thyroplasty in patients who do not have return of vocal cord mobility. The procedure has even been shown to be safe in neonates. Ayoub and colleagues demonstrated the safety and efficacy of injection laryngoplasty in patients aged less than 1 year with unilateral vocal cord paresis reporting improvement in objective swallow function in 89% of patients.[15]

Laryngeal cleft

Laryngeal clefts are communications between the larynx and/or tracheal with the pharynx and/or esophagus. Early in development in utero, the posterior cricoid fuses and the tracheoesophageal septum arises from the foregut at the carina. The septum extends cranially to divide the future larynx and trachea from the esophagus and pharynx. Failure or disruption of this process results in a tracheoesophageal cleft.

Laryngeal clefts are commonly classified as type 1 through type 4 based on the Benjamin–Inglis classification.[16] Type 1 cleft is a deep interarytenoid groove and cleft to the level of the cricoid cartilage. Clefts extending into but not through the cricoid cartilage are classified as type 2. Type 3 clefts extend through the cricoid cartilage and into the trachea. Type 4 clefts involve and significant portion of the trachea and extend to the thoracic trachea. More recent refinements of this classification have included deep interarytenoid grooves. This includes an interarytenoid mucosal defect that does not meet full criteria for a type 1 laryngeal cleft. Definition of a deep interarytenoid groove varies. For example, Wineski and colleagues defined a deep interarytenoid groove as a defect extending to the level of the ventricles.[17] Others describe it as a depression 0 to 3 mm above the vocal cords.[18,19]

Patients with laryngeal clefts present with respiratory symptoms, often exacerbated by feeding. Symptoms range from chronic cough to respiratory distress and cyanosis. Cough, stridor, and respiratory compromise with feeding occur because aspiration is present in patients with tracheoesophageal clefts. Symptoms may also occur in the absence of feeding due to aspiration of saliva. Recurrent pneumonias and pulmonary disease can result from persistent, chronic aspiration. The severity of symptoms will correlate with the severity or type of cleft. Age at presentation and diagnostic evaluation will often correlate with severity of cleft as well. Patients with severe symptoms are more likely to present at an earlier age. Stridor and cyanosis as presenting symptoms are more common in patients aged 0 to 3 months.[20] VFSS or FEES may be suggested for an initial evaluation in patients based on the presenting symptoms. Often, in cases of laryngeal clefts VFSS or FEES will reveal aspiration, but not always. Direct laryngoscopy with close examination and palpation of the posterior larynx is gold standard for diagnosis.

Treatment of a laryngeal cleft is dependent on cleft severity. Deep interarytenoid grooves and type 1 clefts can be managed conservatively with dietary modifications, swallowing therapy, and medications for GERD. Alternatively, an interarytenoid injection or an endoscopic closure of the cleft is surgical option. Endoscopic closure involves denuding the cleft mucosa with cold dissection, coblation or laser, and reapproximating the cleft with sutures. Injection involves interarytenoid injection with an injectable material. Wineski and colleagues showed that addressing the cleft with an injection or endoscopic closure significantly improved postoperative aspiration in patients as compared to conservative management.[17]

Type 2 and some type 3 clefts are amenable to endoscopic repair. Some type 3 and all type 4 clefts typically require an open anterior and/or posterior lateral approach for repair. The majority of patients have improvement in dysphagia after cleft repair. However, the degree of improvement and time to improvement varies given the multifactorial nature of dysphagia.

SUMMARY

Anatomic laryngotracheal abnormalities are closely associated with dysphagia and swallowing dysfunction. They can interfere with the suck–swallow–breathe mechanism and can alter the pharyngeal phase of swallowing. They can lead to respiratory distress or chronic aspiration. Surgical treatment of these anomalies can contribute to or improve swallowing dysfunction. Treatment of patients with laryngotracheal anomalies requires a multidisciplinary approach.

CLINICS CARE POINTS

- Clinical assessment of swallowing function should be performed in patients with symptoms and considered for all patients with laryngomalacia even in the absence of dysphagia symptoms.
- Dysphagia should be assessed postoperatively in patients undergoing supraglottoplasty regardless of preoperative symptoms with special attention during the immediate postoperative period.

- Infants with severe airway obstruction can have difficulty with the suck–swallow–breathe sequence, resulting in dysphagia and even failure to tolerate oral nutrition.
- Injection laryngoplasty may allow initiation of an oral diet or advancement of a previously restricted diet in pediatric patients with vocal cord paralysis. The procedure is associated with a low rate of complications and has been shown to be safe in infants.
- Direct laryngoscopy with close examination and palpation of the posterior larynx is gold standard for the diagnosis of a laryngeal cleft or deep interarytenoid groove contributing to aspiration.
- Injection or endoscopic closure of a cleft or deep interarytenoid groove improves postoperative aspiration in patients as compared to conservative management.

DISCLOSURE

The authors have no financial disclosures.

REFERENCES

1. Richter GT, Wootten CT, Rutter MJ, et al. Impact of supraglottoplasty on aspiration in severe laryngomalacia. Ann Otol Rhinol Laryngol 2009;118(4):259–66.
2. Simons JP, Greenberg LL, Mehta DK, et al. Laryngomalacia and swallowing function in children. Laryngoscope 2016;126(2):478–84.
3. Irace AL, Dombrowski ND, Kawai K, et al. Evaluation of aspiration in infants with laryngomalacia and recurrent respiratory and feeding difficulties. JAMA Otolaryngol Head Neck Surg 2019;145(2):146–51.
4. Nguyen M, Brooks L, Wetzel M, et al. swallowing outcomes following supraglottoplasty: a retrospective review. Laryngoscope 2021 Dec;131(12):2817–22.
5. Myer CM, O'Connor DM, Cotton RT. proposed grading system for subglottic stenosis based on endotracheal tube sizes. Ann Otol Rhinol Laryngol 1994;103:319–23.
6. Cohen SR. Congenital glottic webs in children. Ann Otol Laryngol 1985;94(Suppl 121):1–16.
7. Kou YF, Redmann A, Tabangin ME, et al. Airway and swallowing outcomes following laryngotracheoplasty with posterior grafting in children. Laryngoscope 2021;131:2798–804.
8. Miller CK, Linck J, Willging JP. Duration and extent of dysphagia following pediatric airway reconstruction. Int J Pediatr Otorhinolaryngol 2009;73:573–9.
9. Irace AL, Dombrowski ND, Kawai K, et al. Aspiration in children with unilateral vocal fold paralysis. Laryngoscope 2019;129:569–73.
10. Lesnik M, Thierry B, Blanchard M, et al. Idiopathic bilateral vocal cord paralysis in infants: Case series and literature review. Laryngoscope 2015;125:1724–8.
11. Miyamoto RC, Parikh SR, Gellad W, et al. bilateral congenital vocal cord paralysis: a 16-year institutional review. Otolaryngology-head and neck surgery 2005;133:241–5.
12. Hsu J, Tibbetts KM, Wu D, et al. Swallowing function in pediatric patients with bilateral vocal fold immobility. Int J Pediatr Otorhinolaryngol 2017;93:37–41.
13. Tibbetts KM, Wu D, Hsu JV, et al. Etiology and long-term functional swallow outcomes in pediatric unilateral vocal fold immobility. Int J Pediatr Otorhinolaryngol 2016;88:179–83.

14. Meister KD, Johnson A, Sidell DR. Injection Laryngoplasty for children with unilateral vocal fold paralysis: procedural limitations and swallow outcomes. Otolaryngology-head and neck surgery 2019;160:540–5.
15. Ayoub N, Balakrishnan K, Meister K, et al. Safety and effectiveness of vocal fold injection laryngoplasty in infants less than one year of age. Int J Pediatr Otorhinolaryngol 2023 May;168:111542.
16. Benjamin B, Inglis A. Minor Congenital Laryngeal Clefts: Diagnosis and Classification. Ann Otol Rhinol Laryngol 1989;98:417–20.
17. Wineski RE, Panico E, Karas A, et al. Optimal timing and technique for endoscopic management of dysphagia in pediatric aerodigestive patients. Int J Pediatr Otorhinolaryngol 2021;150:110874.
18. Bakthavachalam S, Schroeder JW, Holinger LD. Diagnosis and management of type I posterior laryngeal clefts. Ann Otol Rhinol Laryngol 2010;119:239–48.
19. Jefferson ND, Carmel E, Cheng ATL. Low inter-arytenoid height: A subclassification of type 1 laryngeal cleft diagnosis and management. Int J Pediatr Otorhinolaryngol 2015;79:31–5.
20. Cole E, Dreyzin A, Shaffer AD, et al. Outcomes and swallowing evaluations after injection laryngoplasty for type I laryngeal cleft: Does age matter? Int J Pediatr Otorhinolaryngol 2018;115:10–8.

Esophageal Dysphagia in Adults: When It Sticks

Miller Richmond, MPH, MD[a], Elliana Kirsh DeVore, MD[b,c],
Phillip C. Song, MD[b,c],*

KEYWORDS

- Esophageal dysphagia • Swallowing difficulty • Adult dysphagia

KEY POINTS

- A proper history and physical examination, including in-office flexible endoscopic examination, can generally determine esophageal versus oropharyngeal dysphagia and subsequent workup.
- Symptoms of dysphagia are difficult to localize, and esophageal pathology often presents in the throat.
- Clinicians should be aware that commonly prescribed medications, including newer drugs such as glucagon-like peptide-1 agonists, can cause dysphagia symptoms.
- Patients with persistent symptoms should have objective testing such as esophagogastroduodenoscopy and barium swallow if not responsive to therapeutic trials.
- Newer diagnosis and treatment modalities such as functional lumen imaging probe and peroral endoscopic myotomy should be considered where available, especially as more supporting data become available.

INTRODUCTION

Esophageal dysphagia is characterized as difficulty swallowing distal to the oropharynx (esophagus, the lower esophageal sphincter [LES], or cardia) due to a structural or functional abnormality. It can also be defined as dysphagia occurring a few seconds after swallowing in patients who have difficulty localizing the sensation. This may manifest as a wide variety of presenting symptoms, including a sensation of food being stuck in the throat, heartburn, halitosis, chest pain, cough, odynophagia, or globus. Esophageal dysphagia significantly impacts quality of life for both patients and caregivers and may devolve into a life-threatening cycle of weight loss, malnutrition, and aspiration, leading to immune deficiency and pneumonia. Dysphagia is prevalent

[a] Georgetown School of Medicine, 3900 Reservoir Road, NW, Washington, DC 20057, USA;
[b] Department of Otolaryngology, Harvard Medical School, 25 Shattuck Street, Boston, MA 02115, USA; [c] Division of Laryngology, Massachusetts Eye and Ear Infirmary, 243 Charles Street, Boston, MA 02114, USA
* Corresponding author.
E-mail address: Phillip_Song@MEEI.HARVARD.EDU

Otolaryngol Clin N Am 57 (2024) 569–579
https://doi.org/10.1016/j.otc.2024.02.027

among Americans, with about 1 in 6 US adults reporting difficulty swallowing, leading to over 860,000 ambulatory office visits and 43,000 emergency department visits for dysphagia annually.[1,2]

Dysphagia more broadly can be particularly dangerous for populations often treated by otolaryngologists, such as elderly individuals and patients with head and neck cancer. Newer chemoradiation and less invasive surgical procedures have failed to decrease dysphagia among patients with head and neck cancer. Instead, research shows an 11% increase in dysphagia when comparing the years 1992 to 1999 to 2002 to 2011. The estimated prevalence among this population at 2 years is 45%, with higher aspiration pneumonia rates than the general population.[3] Estimates of dysphagia prevalence among the general population 65 years of age and older are as high as 40%.[4] Individuals living with dementia or a previous stroke have even higher rates of dysphagia. Pneumonia (likely caused by dysphagia and subsequent aspiration) is estimated to cause 35% of poststroke deaths.[5] Both head and neck cancer and elderly patients can become caught in a vicious cycle of dysphagia, subsequent weight loss/malnutrition, immune system compromise, and aspiration pneumonia.[6] This can lead to increased morbidity/mortality, reduced quality of life, and increased utilization of resources.

Esophageal dysphagia can arise from various etiologies, broadly categorized into 3 major groups: neurologic disorders, esophageal motility disorders, and structural abnormalities. Neurologic disorders such as stroke, neuromuscular disease, myopathy, Parkinson's disease, and amyotrophic lateral sclerosis can affect the nerves and muscles involved in swallowing, leading to dysphagia. Esophageal motility disorders, including achalasia, esophageal spasm, and ineffective esophageal motility (IEM), disrupt the coordinated muscle contractions necessary for propelling food down the esophagus, causing difficulty in swallowing. Structural abnormalities, whether esophageal inflammation or anatomic obstruction, such as esophagitis, esophageal strictures, tumors, and Zenker's diverticulum, can physically narrow or block the esophageal lumen, resulting in dysphagia.

Risk factors for esophageal dysphagia are similar to oropharyngeal dysphagia. Age appears to play a role, with prevalence rising significantly among individuals over 60 years. Additionally, female individuals are at a higher risk compared to male individuals. Certain medical conditions, such as the aforementioned neurologic disorders, gastroesophageal reflux disease (GERD), and head and neck cancers, significantly predispose individuals to esophageal dysphagia. Smoking, alcohol consumption, and poor diet can contribute to esophageal problems and ultimately lead to dysphagia.

DISCUSSION
Clinical Presentation

A patient presenting with esophageal dysphagia typically reports a sensation of a food bolus "sticking" or transiting slowly through the esophagus. Other reported symptoms may include chest pain, weight loss, food impaction, nocturnal regurgitation, reflux, heartburn, or coughing/choking. Some studies show that patients often struggle to localize the issue or differentiate it from oropharyngeal dysphagia. It is not uncommon for patients to report both oropharyngeal and esophageal concerns.[5,7–9] Patients reporting suprasternal pain with swallowing may have referred pain from a more distal site.[10] Overlapping GERD and oropharyngeal dysphagia can make the initial presentation challenging, but a systematic approach to the history and physical will elucidate esophageal dysphagia in most instances.

Evaluation

Esophageal dysphagia workup is a multidisciplinary process involving specialists from gastroenterology, otolaryngology, and speech–language pathology. The initial workup should prioritize a thorough history and physical examination. **Fig. 1** provides an approach to building a differential diagnosis based on clinical history.[11] It is helpful to identify whether symptoms occur with only solid foods or liquids (ie, mixed dysphagia). Specific attention should be paid to the nature of the dysphagia, whether it is progressive, intermittent, or associated with pain. The presence of systemic symptoms such as weight loss or anemia may indicate malignancy. Concurrent allergic rhinitis, asthma, eczema, and other history of atopy may suggest a diagnosis of eosinophilic esophagitis (EoE).[12] Clinicians should ask about any history of surgery or radiation to the head, neck, or spine, xerostomia, food allergies, and acid reflux (and any trials of acid suppression). Neuromuscular disease may manifest in both oropharyngeal and esophageal dysphagia.[13] Additional risk factors include diabetes, alcoholism, and neuropathy. Finally, commonly used medications, as listed in **Fig. 2**, can cause either pill-induced esophagitis by direct damage to the esophageal lining or esophageal motility issues by impaired relaxation in the LES.[14,15] The increasingly popular glucagon-like peptide-1 receptor (GLP-1) agonists such as semaglutide and tirzepatide cause delayed gastric emptying, which can lead to the development of dysphagia, GERD, and gastrointestinal distress.[16–18]

Patient-reported outcome measures (PROMs) are commonly used to capture patient experience with dysphagia and to evaluate the effect of treatments. Validated instruments exist for the evaluation of general dysphagia, such as the NIH Patient-Reported Outcomes Measurement Information System gastrointestinal symptom scale.[19] In addition, there are several high-quality measures for specific conditions, such as achalasia, Parkinson's disease, EoE, and esophageal cancer.[20–23] Of note, dysphagia-related PROMs demonstrated significant variability in their developmental

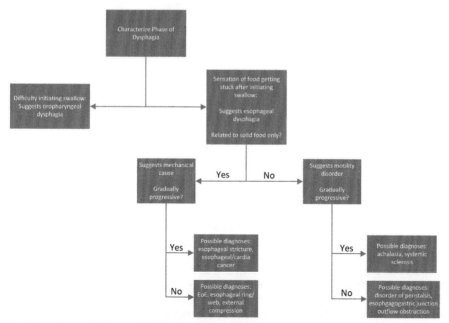

Fig. 1. Differential diagnosis of dysphagia in adults.

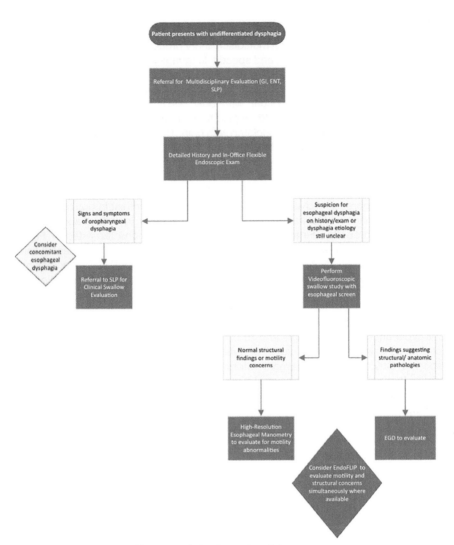

Fig. 2. Evaluation of undifferentiated dysphagia in adults.

rigor, with several failing to establish responsiveness to change for longitudinal symptom assessment or involving insufficient input from patients during content conception.[24] Nevertheless, several robust measures are available for use in clinical practice to understand patients' perception of how the disease is affecting their quality of life.

For the otolaryngologist, the initial physical examination often involves an in-office flexible endoscopic evaluation. This examination is crucial for ruling out oropharyngeal dysphagia and identifying features of laryngopharyngeal reflux (LPR). LPR features, such as redness or swelling in the throat and larynx, might coexist with or contribute to esophageal dysphagia. Additionally, this examination can reveal the pooling of secretions, which might indicate swallowing dysfunction. The flexible endoscopic examination provides a detailed assessment of the oropharyngeal swallow and offers insight into potential esophageal issues.

Any patient without a clear oropharyngeal cause for their dysphagia should undergo a video fluoroscopic swallow study (VFSS) with esophageal screen to identify distal abnormalities. Compared to a comprehensive video fluoroscopic esophagram, VFSS with ES has a sensitivity of 63% and specificity of 100%.[25] In general, patients are more sensitive to their symptoms than testing. Refer to the chapter by Dr Bryson for more information regarding swallow studies.

For individuals noted to have a structural or anatomic pathology or concern for mucosal abnormality, an esophagogastroduodenoscopy (EGD) is utilized to view the esophageal lumen and obtain biopsy of any suspicious lesions. Up to 64% of patients with motility disorders will also have an abnormal EGD, making it a useful adjunct to high-resolution esophageal manometry (HRM).[26] Tracking resistance in the esophagogastric junction (EGJ), residue in the lumen, and contraction during EGD can help elicit some of these abnormalities. EGDs also have therapeutic capabilities, such as dilation, which can provide the patient with some relief.[27] Lastly, EGDs can be cost-effective screening tools for patients found to have benign structural pathologies.[28]

If these studies are unrevealing or a motility disorder is suspected based on patient history, HRM continues to be the gold standard for nonobstructive dysphagia.[29] Esophageal manometry utilizes a pressure-sensing catheter inserted into the esophagus while an awake patient sips water. Measurements taken include the integrated relaxation pressure, esophageal contractility, pressurization, and timing of contractions with deglutition.[30] These results are interpreted according to the Chicago Classification, allowing for objective analysis of HRM metrics and topography, as well as prognostication of disease.[31]

Individuals may have LPR as an underlying cause to their dysphagia.[32] Dual pH studies may be helpful in diagnosis and management for patients whose symptoms are refractive to empirical acid suppression, whereby a probe is placed above the upper esophageal sphincter to measure acidic events.[33,34] Oropharyngeal pH monitoring, such as the ResTech Device (Respiratory Technology Corporation, Houston, Texas), is useful in detecting hypopharyngeal reflux events (HREs) by measuring aerosolized acidic vapor. The composite score of the Restech measurement, the RYAN score, is a derivative of the DeMeester score and useful in identifying abnormal acid exposure. Hypopharyngeal–esophageal multichannel intraluminal impedance-pH monitoring detects pH and intraesophageal bolus movement by measuring the change in resistance to current flow between 2 electrodes with a liquid or gas bolus bridges. This testing describes the type and composition of HRE and the LPR features. In sum, further objective examination to confirm diagnosis may be pursued for patients unresponsive to empirical therapeutic trial for LPR.

A combination of endoscopy and manometry is functional lumen imaging probe (FLIP) or "Endoflip." This is a newer technique that can be performed during upper endoscopy while a patient is sedated.[35] It also consists of a pressure-sensing catheter inserted into the esophagus, but the swallowing function is mimicked by filling the catheter with saline. Two primary measurements are provided in FLIP evaluation: the EGI-distensibility index (EGJ-DI) and FLIP panometry. EGJ-DI calculates the flexibility of the sphincter by dividing the average smallest cross-sectional area by the average pressure inside the balloon over a specific period.[36] Pathology is suspected with an EGJ-DI less than 2 mm^2/mm Hg or an EGJ diameter of less than 13 mm.[37] FLIP panometry measures esophageal motility by inducing distension along the esophagus and has recently been shown to possibly be equivalent to HRM.[38] FLIP, combined with upper endoscopy, can provide a structural and motility assessment in one procedure with the patient sedated, improving efficiency and patient comfort. However, more data are needed to confirm its role beyond a complementary tool to the gold standard of HRM.[36,39]

DIFFERENTIAL DIAGNOSIS

The first objective when formulating a differential diagnosis for patients' symptoms is to distinguish between motility disorders versus anatomic or structural etiologies. Infectious causes of dysphagia should also be considered. Functional dysphagia remains a diagnosis of exclusion.

Motility Pathologies

Intermittent symptoms of long duration, occurring with both solids and liquids, are more indicative of motility disorders. The Chicago Classification system allows for manometric findings to separate motility disorders into 2 main categories: esophagogastric junction outflow obstruction (EGJOO) and disorders of peristalsis.[30] EGJOO can be associated with achalasia or a structural cause within the esophagus can cause abnormal findings. Achalasia is a common disorder of motility that combines both categories, consisting of impaired relaxation of the LES and abnormal peristalsis in the esophagus.

Motility disorders can also be separated into abnormalities of inhibitory innervation and excitatory/smooth muscle innervation. Achalasia and distal/diffuse esophageal spasm (DES) are a result of decreased inhibition. Increased inhibition can lead to over-relaxation of the LES resulting in acid reflux-related motility problems. Excitatory and smooth muscle innervation issues can lead to "hypotensive" (seen in scleroderma, hypotensive LES, and IEM disease) and "hypertensive" (such as jackhammer esophagus and hypertensive LES). There is often overlap in pathologies. More common, nonmotility-related, causes of dysphagia affecting the patient can also be found despite positive findings on manometry. Lastly, DES and jackhammer esophagus, in particular, can present similar to the chest pain of cardiac origin. Patients with risk factors for cardiac angina should undergo a workup with a cardiologist.[40] Given this complexity, clinicians must allocate appropriate resources for accurate diagnosis of motility pathologies and be vigilant of other possible diagnoses.

Structural and Anatomic Pathologies

Esophageal dysphagia symptoms can be caused by structural abnormalities, including cricopharyngeal dysfunction, diverticula, and hiatal hernias. Anatomic esophageal obstruction can occur intrinsically via strictures, rings, and webs and extrinsically through vascular compression, a substernal thyroid, mediastinal lymphadenopathy, and tumors. Peptic strictures often arise from chronic GERD, causing progressive dysphagia.[41] Schatzki rings, associated with hiatal hernias, typically manifest as intermittent dysphagia for solid foods.[42] Additionally, benign and malignant tumors can lead to progressive dysphagia. For this reason, esophageal cancer should be an early consideration, given malignancy is associated with high mortality. Long-standing or severe esophagitis can lead to the development of intrinsic obstructions such as strictures and rings. Caustic esophagitis from ingesting corrosive substances may also result in severe mucosal damage and strictures.

Infectious and Inflammatory Etiologies

Various causes of inflammation within the esophagus, or esophagitis, commonly cause esophageal dysphagia. Reflux esophagitis is caused by chronic GERD, leading to irritation and inflammation. Another uncommon inflammatory etiology is EoE, an allergic condition marked by eosinophil infiltration in the esophagus on biopsy; EoE can mimic the symptoms of GERD but typically shows resistance to standard acid-suppressive therapy. The current incidence of EoE is estimated at 5 to 10 cases per 100,000, higher in high-income countries, male individuals, and North America (vs Europe and Asia).[43] Infectious esophagitis is common in immunocompromised patients and can be caused by fungi, viruses, or bacteria, leading to severe pain, ulceration, and narrowing of the esophagus. Drug-induced esophagitis (**Table 1**) can occur due to improper administration of certain medications, when not taken properly, and can cause direct irritation to the esophagus.

MANAGEMENT
Management of Motility Disorders

Motility disorders can be challenging to treat. Hypercontractile disorders, such as DES and jackhammer esophagus, are generally treated with medications. Smooth muscle relaxants such as nitrates, calcium channel blockers, and peppermint oil can be used to relax the esophageal muscles.[44,45] However, underlying or undertreated GERD can be exacerbated by smooth muscle relaxants, and patients should be followed closely. tricyclic antidepressants (TCAs), trazodone, sildenafil, and selective serotonin reuptake inhibitors (SSRIs) can be used to reduce the sensitivity of the esophagus.[45] Additionally, biofeedback and cognitive behavioral therapy have shown some positive results for some patients. Heller myotomy and peroral endoscopic myotomy (POEM) are more invasive but can be options after medical management has failed. IEM should be managed with small meals, avoiding laying down after eating, and occasionally prokinetic medications. Underlying GERD should be treated aggressively in all patients with motility disorders.

Most treatment options for achalasia focus on symptom management and relaxation of the LES. Treatment plans for patients will be determined by an individual's age, surgical risk, degree of impairment, and the expertise of the clinician. First-line endoscopic treatment with pneumatic dilation improves symptoms in many patients. Some patients can even tolerate this in the office.[40,46] Heller myotomy is generally done laparoscopically and is a more definitive treatment option. Where available, POEM is a largely safe endoscopic treatment option with similar success rates as the Heller myotomy. These procedures carry potential complications such as perforation and worsening of GERD.[47,48] Patients who are not healthy enough to tolerate more invasive options often see benefits from endoscopic botulinum toxin injection of the LES.[46] Finally, patients on chronic opioids will continue to be refractory to most treatments without moving to non-narcotic pain relievers.

Table 1	
Common medications implicated in esophageal dysphagia	
Pill Esophagitis	**Esophageal Motility**
Nonsteroidal anti-inflammatory drugs	Nitrates
Tetracyclines	Anticholinergics
Potassium chloride	Benzodiazepines
Quinidine	Opioids
Ferrous sulfate	Calcium channel blockers
Ascorbic acid	Tricyclic antidepressants
	GLP-1 agonists (semaglutide)

Management of Structural and Anatomic Pathologies

Hiatal hernias, esophageal diverticula, and extrinsic compression of the esophagus should address the underlying cause directly if possible. Intrinsic pathologies, such as webs, strictures, and rings, are often caused by reflux, leading to the initial treatments of esophageal dilation and acid suppression. Dilation is widely regarded as generally safe and effective, and long-term acid suppression helps prevent recurrence.[49] Risks include perforation or bleeding from dilation, and the effect of long-term acid suppression with proton-pump inhibitors (PPIs) continues to be studied.[50] When needed, endoscopic management of intrinsic obstructions can be done with needle knife incision, stents, or steroid injections as needed.[40]

Management of Esophagitis

Management of EoE and other inflammatory esophageal conditions primarily involves dietary modifications, pharmacologic therapy, and endoscopic interventions to alleviate symptoms and control inflammation. Dietary strategies often include elimination diets where common allergens are removed and gradually reintroduced to identify triggers. Topical corticosteroids, such as fluticasone or budesonide, are frequently prescribed to reduce esophageal inflammation and prevent stricture formation. PPI may be employed for both acid suppression and potential anti-inflammatory effects.[40] In cases where strictures have developed, esophageal dilation might be performed to relieve dysphagia. The management approach is usually tailored to the individual's response to treatment and is often a collaborative effort alongside allergists and dietitians. Regular monitoring through endoscopy and biopsies is crucial to assess treatment effectiveness and make necessary adjustments, aiming for both symptomatic relief and histologic remission.

Pill-induced esophagitis and other caustic damage to the esophagus are generally managed with the removal of the offending agent coupled with short-term acid suppression and sucralfate to allow healing of the ulcer.[51] Endoscopy should only be repeated if symptoms do not improve after sufficient time for healing.[52] Infectious esophagitis care should include an immunocompetency workup (with treatment as necessary) in addition to treatment of the organism.

In all these scenarios, the importance of individualized treatment plans and regular follow-ups cannot be overstated. Interdisciplinary care is vital for managing complex cases and ensuring the best outcomes for patients facing a spectrum of esophageal conditions. Each treatment strategy should be considered within the broader context of the patient's overall health, response to previous treatments, and potential for complications.

CLINICS CARE POINTS

- Patients younger than 50 years with dysphagia, no risk factors, and no alarm symptoms may try an oral PPI with close interval follow-up.

- Endoscopy with biopsy is preferred for evaluation of structural, inflammatory, and neoplastic findings.

- Individuals determined to have a motility disorder by history or inconclusive endoscopy/ esophogram study should undergo high-resolution manometry.

- First-line treatment of achalasia for generally healthy patients is endoscopic or surgical management. Medical management should be attempted with other motility disorders.

- FLIP is a newer tool that allows for motility evaluation during the initial endoscopy and should be considered where available and when there is suspicion for underlying motility pathology

DISCLOSURE

The authors have nothing to disclose.

REFERENCES

1. Adkins C, Takakura W, Spiegel BMR, et al. Prevalence and characteristics of dysphagia based on a population-based survey. Clin Gastroenterol Hepatol 2020;18(9):1970–9.e2.
2. Peery AF, Crockett SD, Murphy CC, et al. Burden and cost of gastrointestinal, liver, and pancreatic diseases in the united states: update 2018. Gastroenterology 2019;156(1):254–72.e11.
3. Hutcheson KA, Nurgalieva Z, Zhao H, et al. Two-year prevalence of dysphagia and related outcomes in head and neck cancer survivors: An updated SEER-Medicare analysis. Head Neck 2019;41(2):479–87.
4. Rofes L, Arreola V, Almirall J, et al. Diagnosis and management of oropharyngeal dysphagia and its nutritional and respiratory complications in the elderly. Gastroenterol Res Pract 2011;2011:1–13.
5. Crary M, Sura L, Madhavan A, et al. Dysphagia in the elderly: management and nutritional considerations. Clin Interv Aging 2012;287. https://doi.org/10.2147/CIA.S23404.
6. Gorenc M, Kozjek NR, Strojan P. Malnutrition and cachexia in patients with head and neck cancer treated with (chemo)radiotherapy. Rep Pract Oncol Radiother 2015;20(4):249–58.
7. Roeder BE, Murray JA, Dierkhising RA. Patient Localization of Esophageal Dysphagia. Dig Dis Sci 2004;49(4):697–701.
8. Ashraf HH, Palmer J, Dalton HR, et al. Can patients determine the level of their dysphagia? World J Gastroenterol 2017;23(6):1038–43.
9. Gullung JL, Hill EG, Castell DO, et al. Oropharyngeal and esophageal swallowing impairments: their association and the predictive value of the modified barium swallow impairment profile and combined multichannel intraluminal impedance—esophageal manometry. Ann Otol Rhinol Laryngol 2012;121(11):738–45.
10. Mel Wilcox C, Alexander LN, Scott Clark W. Localization of an obstructing esophageal lesion: Is the patient accurate? Dig Dis Sci 1995;40(10):2192–6.
11. Dickman R, Mattek N, Holub J, et al. Prevalence of upper gastrointestinal tract findings in patients with noncardiac chest pain versus those with gastroesophageal reflux disease (GERD)-related symptoms: results from a national endoscopic database. Am J Gastroenterol 2007;102(6):1173–9.
12. Simon HU, Straumann A. Immunopathogenesis of eosinophilic esophagitis. Dig Dis 2014;32(1–2):11–4.
13. Hurtte E, Young J, Gyawali CP. Dysphagia. Prim Care Clin 2023;50(3):325–38.
14. Wilkinson JM, Halland M. Esophageal motility disorders. Am Fam Physician 2020; 102(5):291–6.
15. Kraichely RE, Arora AS, Murray JA. Opiate-induced oesophageal dysmotility. Aliment Pharmacol Ther 2010;31(5):601–6.
16. Nakatani Y, Maeda M, Matsumura M, et al. Effect of GLP-1 receptor agonist on gastrointestinal tract motility and residue rates as evaluated by capsule endoscopy. Diabetes Metab 2017;43(5):430–7.
17. Quast DR, Schenker N, Menge BA, et al. Effects of lixisenatide versus liraglutide (short- and long-acting GLP-1 receptor agonists) on esophageal and gastric function in patients with type 2 diabetes. Diabetes Care 2020;43(9):2137–45.

18. Liu BD, Udemba SC, Liang K, et al. Shorter-acting glucagon-like peptide-1 receptor agonists are associated with increased development of gastro-oesophageal reflux disease and its complications in patients with type 2 diabetes mellitus: a population-level retrospective matched cohort study. Gut 2023;73(2):246–54.

19. Spiegel BMR, Hays RD, Bolus R, et al. Development of the NIH patient-reported outcomes measurement information system (PROMIS) gastrointestinal symptom scales. Am J Gastroenterol 2014;109(11):1804–14.

20. Urbach DR, Tomlinson GA, Harnish JL, et al. A measure of disease-specific health-related quality of life for achalasia. Am J Gastroenterol 2005;100(8):1668–76.

21. Chen AY, Frankowski R, Bishop-Leone J, et al. The development and validation of a dysphagia-specific quality-of-life questionnaire for patients with head and neck cancer: the M. D. Anderson dysphagia inventory. Arch Otolaryngol Head Neck Surg 2001;127(7):870–6.

22. Dellon ES, Irani AM, Hill MR, et al. Development and field testing of a novel patient-reported outcome measure of dysphagia in patients with eosinophilic esophagitis. Aliment Pharmacol Ther 2013;38(6):634–42.

23. Lagergren P, Fayers P, Conroy T, et al. Clinical and psychometric validation of a questionnaire module, the EORTC QLQ-OG25, to assess health-related quality of life in patients with cancer of the oesophagus, the oesophago–gastric junction and the stomach. Eur J Cancer 2007;43(14):2066–73.

24. Patel DA, Sharda R, Hovis KL, et al. Patient-reported outcome measures in dysphagia: a systematic review of instrument development and validation. Dis Esophagus 2017;30(5):1–23.

25. Belafsky PC, Kuhn MA. The clinician's guide to swallowing fluoroscopy. New York: Springer; 2014.

26. Matsubara M, Manabe N, Ayaki M, et al. Clinical significance of esophagogastro-duodenoscopy in patients with esophageal motility disorders. Dig Endosc 2021;33(5):753–60.

27. Pasha SF, Acosta RD, Chandrasekhara V, et al. The role of endoscopy in the evaluation and management of dysphagia. Gastrointest Endosc 2014;79(2):191–201.

28. Esfandyari T, Potter JW, Vaezi MF. Dysphagia: a cost analysis of the diagnostic approach. Am J Gastroenterol 2002;97(11):2733–7.

29. Carlson DA, Pandolfino JE. High-resolution manometry in clinical practice. Gastroenterol Hepatol 2015;11(6):374–84.

30. Yadlapati R, Kahrilas PJ, Fox MR, et al. Esophageal motility disorders on high-resolution manometry: Chicago classification version 4.0©. Neuro Gastroenterol Motil 2021;33(1):e14058.

31. Rohof WOA, Bredenoord AJ. Chicago classification of esophageal motility disorders: lessons learned. Curr Gastroenterol Rep 2017;19(8):37.

32. Bobin F, Lechien JR. The role of pH-impedance monitoring in swallowing disorders. Curr Opin Otolaryngol Head Neck Surg 2022;30(6):406–16.

33. Vance D, Park J, Alnouri G, et al. Diagnosing laryngopharyngeal reflux: a comparison between 24-hour pH-impedance testing and pharyngeal probe (Restech) testing, with introduction of the Sataloff score. J Voice 2023;37(5):737–47.

34. Babic B, Müller DT, Gebauer F, et al. Gastrointestinal function testing model using a new laryngopharyngeal pH probe (Restech) in patients after Ivor-Lewis esophagectomy. World J Gastrointest Oncol 2021;13(6):612–24.

35. Carlson DA, Kahrilas PJ, Lin Z, et al. Evaluation of esophageal motility utilizing the functional lumen imaging probe. Am J Gastroenterol 2016;111(12):1726–35.

36. Donnan EN, Pandolfino JE. Endoflip in the esophagus. Gastroenterol Clin North Am 2020;49(3):427–35.
37. Patel DA, Yadlapati R, Vaezi MF. Esophageal motility disorders: current approach to diagnostics and therapeutics. Gastroenterology 2022;162(6):1617–34.
38. Carlson DA, Gyawali CP, Khan A, et al. Classifying esophageal motility by FLIP panometry: a study of 722 subjects with manometry. Am J Gastroenterol 2021; 116(12):2357–66.
39. Hirano I, Pandolfino JE, Boeckxstaens GE. Functional lumen imaging probe for the management of esophageal disorders: expert review from the clinical practice updates committee of the AGA institute. Clin Gastroenterol Hepatol 2017;15(3):325–34.
40. Lynch KL, Katzka DA. Dysphagia: how to recognize and narrow the differential. In: Patel DA, Kavitt RT, Vaezi MF, editors. Evaluation and management of dysphagia. Switzerland: Springer International Publishing; 2020. p. 1–12.
41. Richter JE. Peptic strictures of the esophagus. Gastroenterol Clin North Am 1999; 28(4):875–91.
42. Müller M, Gockel I, Hedwig P, et al. Is the Schatzki ring a unique esophageal entity? World J Gastroenterol 2011;17(23):2838–43.
43. Hahn JW, Lee K, Shin JI, et al. Global incidence and prevalence of eosinophilic esophagitis, 1976-2022: a systematic review and meta-analysis. Clin Gastroenterol Hepatol 2023;21(13):3270–84.e77.
44. Pimentel M, Bonorris GG, Chow EJ, et al. Peppermint oil improves the manometric findings in diffuse esophageal spasm. J Clin Gastroenterol 2001;33(1):27–31.
45. Maradey-Romero C, Gabbard S, Fass R. Treatment of esophageal motility disorders based on the Chicago classification. Curr Treat Options Gastroenterol 2014; 12(4):441–55.
46. Wellenstein DJ, Schutte HW, Marres HAM, et al. Office-based procedures for diagnosis and treatment of esophageal pathology. Head Neck 2017;39(9):1910–9.
47. Schlottmann F, Luckett DJ, Fine J, et al. Laparoscopic heller myotomy versus peroral endoscopic myotomy (poem) for achalasia: a systematic review and meta-analysis. Ann Surg 2018;267(3):451–60.
48. Kumbhari V, Familiari P, Bjerregaard N, et al. Gastroesophageal reflux after peroral endoscopic myotomy: a multicenter case–control study. Endoscopy 2017;49(07): 634–42.
49. Liu LWC, Andrews CN, Armstrong D, et al. Clinical practice guidelines for the assessment of uninvestigated esophageal dysphagia. J Can Assoc Gastroenterol 2018;1(1):5–19.
50. Freedberg DE, Kim LS, Yang YX. The risks and benefits of long-term use of proton pump inhibitors: expert review and best practice advice from the American gastroenterological association. Gastroenterology 2017;152(4):706–15.
51. Kim SH, Jeong JB, Kim JW, et al. Clinical and endoscopic characteristics of drug-induced esophagitis. World J Gastroenterol 2014;20(31):10994.
52. Zografos GN, Georgiadou D, Thomas D, et al. Drug-induced esophagitis. Dis Esophagus 2009;22(8):633–7.

Pediatric Esophageal Dysphagia

Erin R.S. Hamersley, DO, CDR, MC, USN[a,b,]*,
Cristina Baldassari, MD, FAAP, FACS[b,c]

KEYWORDS

- Esophageal strictures • Vascular ring • Vascular sling • Esophageal dysphagia

KEY POINTS

- Dysphagia is a common symptom in the pediatric population and is often multifactorial in nature and thus is best managed with a multidisciplinary team.
- Structural causes of esophageal dysphagia in pediatric patients occur secondary to intrinsic pathology or extrinsic compression, resulting in a narrowed esophageal lumen.
- Esophageal stricture is common following tracheoesophageal fistula and esophageal atresia repair but is also seen in the setting of caustic ingestion, eosinophilic esophagitis, and uncontrolled gastroesophageal reflux disease.
- Vascular rings and slings occur as a result of malformation of the primitive aortic arch system and can lead to respiratory and swallowing complaints when they cause compression on the aerodigestive tract.

INTRODUCTION

Swallowing is an intricate process that requires complex coordination of the nervous and muscular systems.[1] The three phases of swallowing (oral, pharyngeal, and esophageal) require voluntary and involuntary neuromuscular contraction in order to successfully move a food bolus from the mouth to the stomach.[1,2] The esophageal phase of swallowing requires relaxation of the upper esophageal sphincter, followed by coordinated smooth muscle peristalsis to propel the bolus through the esophagus, and ends with relaxation of the lower esophageal sphincter to allow the bolus to enter the stomach.[1] The esophagus serves as a conduit from the pharynx to the stomach, thus any type of obstruction to this involuntary movement of the food bolus can lead

[a] Department of Otolaryngology - Head and Neck Surgery, Naval Medical Center Portsmouth, 620 John Paul Jones Cir, Portsmouth, VA, 23708, USA; [b] Department of Otolaryngology - Head and Neck Surgery, Eastern Virginia Medical School, 600 Gresham Drive, Norfolk, VA 23507, USA; [c] Department of Pediatric Sleep Medicine, Children's Hospital of the King's Daughters, 601 Children's Ln, Norfolk, VA 23507, USA
* Corresponding author. Department of Otolaryngology, Sentara, Norfolk General Hospital, 600 Gresham Drive, Norfolk, VA 23507.
E-mail address: erinspadaro@gmail.com

Otolaryngol Clin N Am 57 (2024) 581–587
https://doi.org/10.1016/j.otc.2024.02.015
0030-6665/24/Published by Elsevier Inc.

to dysphagia. Abnormalities within the esophageal phase of swallowing are often grouped broadly into structural and nonstructural. This chapter reviews the structural causes of pediatric esophageal dysphagia focusing on esophageal strictures, vascular rings, and vascular slings.

HISTORY/BACKGROUND

Pediatric dysphagia has an estimated incidence of 0.9% in the general population, although it is higher in at-risk populations including those with a history of prematurity and those with neurologic and cardiorespiratory comorbidities.[2,3] Patient presentations vary depending on the age of the patient and underlying cause of the dysphagia symptoms.[2] The cause of dysphagia is often multifactorial in the pediatric population and thus is best managed with a multidisciplinary team for appropriate diagnosis and treatment. Patients should undergo a complete history and physical examination to better characterize their dysphagia to assist with identifying which phase of swallow may be affected and to uncover any contributing factors and potential associated symptoms (respiratory symptoms, recurrent illnesses, recurrent pneumonias). A pediatric speech and language pathologist should evaluate the patient as part of their initial workup and will assist with their swallow evaluation, which may be completed via flexible endoscopic evaluation of swallowing and/or modified barium swallow, also referred to as videofluoroscopic swallow study.[1,2] When there is concern for a structural esophageal abnormality as the cause for the dysphagia, additional workup should be conducted and may include an esophagram, which is also known as a barium swallow, chest radiograph, echocardiogram, esophagogastroduodenoscopy (EGD), and potentially direct laryngoscopy and rigid bronchoscopy.[1,3,4] Depending on the findings in the aforementioned studies, additional imaging to include chest computed tomography (CT) or magnetic resonance imaging or angiography may be required to better evaluate the vascular system to diagnose a vascular ring or sling.[1,4]

Definitions

- Esophageal stricture: abnormal narrowing of the esophageal lumen
- Vascular ring: congenital abnormality of the aortic arch system that results in compression of the trachea and/or esophagus[4,5]
- Vascular sling: a rare congenital vascular abnormality that occurs when the left pulmonary artery arises from the right pulmonary artery and encircles the right mainstem bronchus and trachea and traverses between the trachea and esophagus before entering the left lung. Vascular slings cause anterior compression of the esophagus.[4,5]
- Dysphagia lusoria: difficulty swallowing secondary to external compression of the esophagus by an aberrant right subclavian artery[2,6]

DISCUSSION

Structural causes of esophageal dysphagia are anatomic abnormalities that narrow the lumen of the esophagus either internally (esophageal strictures) or by external compression (vascular ring or sling). The severity of a patient's symptoms and timing of presentation depend on the severity of the narrowing of the esophagus. Dysphagia from vascular rings and slings is more commonly seen around the time the child begins to eat more solid foods.[5] Patients with esophageal strictures or vascular rings or slings may complain of or demonstrate signs or symptoms of dysphagia, reflux, coughing/choking, or poor weight gain/failure to thrive.[5] Children with vascular rings and slings may also have airway symptoms to include chronic cough, recurrent respiratory illnesses or pneumonias, stridor, or apneic events, thus initial history should include an investigation for these symptoms.[4]

Esophageal strictures may be the result of caustic ingestions, chronic uncontrolled gastroesophageal reflux disease, following tracheoesophageal fistula (TEF) or esophageal atresia (EA) repairs, or rarely a complication of eosinophilic esophagitis.[1] Esophageal stricture following TEF/EA repair is the most common postoperative complication, presenting in as many as 40% to 56% of cases.[7] Stricture formation following TEF/EA repair typically presents within the first 3 months following the procedure.[7] Caustic ingestion may lead to esophageal stricture in 2% to 49% of cases, although the incidence is significantly higher in the setting of severe burns (grades 2b and 3) ranging as high as 77% to 90%, respectively.[8,9] Esophageal strictures may be diagnosed with an esophagram (**Fig. 1**), modified barium swallow, or EGD. Treatment of esophageal strictures generally involves dilation, which was previously commonly completed with bougie dilators, although now it is achieved via balloon dilation (**Fig. 2**A, B).[10] Balloon dilation is favored for its circumferential radial force and elimination of the shearing force that is associated with the use of rigid bougie dilators.[10] Most patients require multiple dilations for successful treatment and symptom mitigation.[10] Caustic strictures can be successfully managed with dilation in 60% to 80% of cases; however, balloon dilation outcomes in the setting of caustic injury have poorer outcomes in

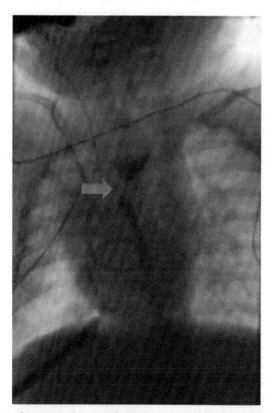

Fig. 1. Esophagram demonstrating esophageal stricture following TEF/EA repair marked with blue arrow.

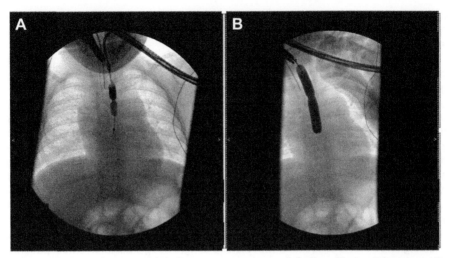

Fig. 2. Esophageal stricture with balloon traversing stenosis before dilation (*A*) and postdilation (*B*).

comparison with alternate causes of stricture formation.[9] Additional treatment adjuncts include intralesional steroid injections and mitomycin-C application. Refractory strictures may require resection and reanastomosis or, in severe cases, esophageal replacement with an interposition graft, although these approaches are at risk for repeat stricture formation with the former and high morbidity rates and uncertain long-term results with the latter.[8]

Aortic arch abnormalities are present in approximately 3% of the population.[4] Vascular rings occur when portions of the primitive aortic arch system persist or fail to regress appropriately.[5] Vascular rings are typically classified as complete (true) rings and incomplete or partial rings. The two complete vascular rings include a double aortic arch and a right aortic arch with an aberrant left subclavian artery and left ligamentum arteriosum.[4,5] Complete rings result in airway and esophageal symptoms. Double aortic arch is the most common vascular ring and the only ring that completely encircles the trachea and esophagus (**Figs. 3** and **4**).[4,5] The circumferential compression

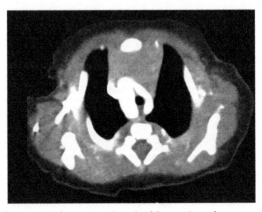

Fig. 3. CT chest with contrast demonstrating double aortic arch.

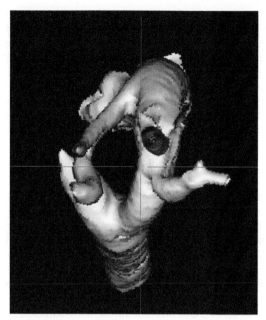

Fig. 4. CT chest with contrast demonstrating 3-dimensional reconstruction of double aortic arch.

around the trachea and esophagus causes symptoms in early infancy including biphasic stridor, recurrent pneumonias, chronic or recurrent lower respiratory infections, wheezing, cyanosis exacerbated by feeding, and less commonly dysphagia.[4] A right aortic arch, left subclavian artery, and left ligamentum arteriosum lead to less compression of the aerodigestive tract, thus these patients typically have a more delayed presentation of their symptoms, typically within the first several years of life.[4,5] Dysphagia in this setting may be more subtle and may present as prolonged times to finish meals.[5]

Vascular slings are caused by malformation of the sixth aortic arch, which leads to a left pulmonary artery originating from the right pulmonary artery and then passes between the trachea and esophagus before inserting into the left lung hilum.[4] The pulmonary artery sling results in compression of the trachea, right mainstem bronchus, and anterior aspect of the esophagus.[4] Complete tracheal rings and long-segment tracheal stenosis are frequently also identified in patients presenting with pulmonary artery slings.[4]

An aberrant right subclavian artery occurs when the origin of the artery arises from the descending thoracic aorta as the final branch of the aortic arch.[4,5] The aberrant right subclavian artery traverses posterior to the esophagus in 80% of cases, splits the esophagus and trachea in 15% of cases, and courses anterior to the trachea or mainstem bronchus in 5% of cases.[6] When a retroesophageal course is present, it causes posterior compression of the esophagus and thus can lead to dysphagia, also referred to as dysphagia lusoria.[4,6] Most patients, however, are asymptomatic.[4]

Diagnostic workup for a vascular ring or sling includes a barium esophagram, which will show an indentation in the esophagus, depending on the underlying anomaly.[4] The diagnosis is then typically confirmed with magnetic resonance angiography to better define the vascular anatomy.[4] An echocardiogram and CT chest with contrast may also assist with diagnosis. When rigid bronchoscopy is performed, a pulsatile compression may be noted in the pattern of the compression associated with the respective anomaly. Additionally, bronchoscopy is valuable to assess the degree of airway impact from the vascular ring or sling to assist with surgical planning. When patients are symptomatic, surgical correction is completed with a cardiothoracic surgeon, which typically eliminates the dysphagia symptoms, although the airway symptoms may persist due to secondary tracheomalacia.[4] Care for these patients can be complex given their constellation of airway and swallowing complaints and thus is best addressed by a multidisciplinary Aerodigestive Team, Cardiology, and Cardiothoracic Surgery.

SUMMARY

Structural pediatric esophageal dysphagia is related to intrinsic or extrinsic factors that narrow the lumen of the esophagus, preventing the involuntary movement of a food bolus from the pharynx into the stomach. A detailed history and evaluation with a multidisciplinary team will help to better guide the initial steps to diagnosis. An esophagram will further assist with identifying a stricture or external compression as the source for the patient's symptoms. Endoscopy and angiography may be required to solidify a final diagnosis. Surgical intervention is often required for structural causes of esophageal dysphagia in the form of balloon dilation or cardiothoracic surgical interventions to improve the caliber of the esophagus and alleviate the symptoms.

CLINICS CARE POINTS

- Diagnosis and management of pediatric patients with esophageal dysphagia should be done in a multidisciplinary setting to include Pediatric Otolaryngology, Gastroenterology, Pulmonology, Radiology, Speech and Language Pathology, Cardiology, and Cardiothoracic Surgery.
- An esophagram should be obtained to identify the location and extent of compression or stenosis of the esophageal lumen.
- Magnetic resonance angiography, an echocardiogram, and potentially a CT of the chest with contrast (depending on the presentation) should be ordered if a vascular ring or sling is suspected.
- Structural causes of esophageal dysphagia are typically managed surgically either through balloon dilation or through cardiothoracic surgical correction of a vascular ring or sling.

DISCLOSURES

Dr E.R.S. Hamersley is a member of the United States Navy. The views expressed in this article reflect the results of research conducted by the author and do not necessarily reflect the official policy or position of the Department of the Navy, Department of Defense, nor the United States Government. "I am a military service member or federal/contracted employee of the United States government. This work was prepared as part of my official duties. Title 17 U.S.C. 105 provides that 'copyright protection under this title is not available for any work of the United States Government.' Title 17 U.S.C. 101 defines a US Government work as work prepared by a military service member or employee of the US Government as part of that person's official duties."

REFERENCES

1. Bromwich M, Cohen A, Miller C, et al. Chapter 74 pediatric dysphagia. In: Bluestone and stool's pediatric otolaryngology. Fifth Edition. People's Medical Publishing House; 2014. p. 1311–21.
2. Moroco AE, Aaronson NL. Pediatric dysphagia. Pediatr Clin North Am 2022; 69(2):349–61.
3. Lawlor CM, Choi S. Diagnosis and management of pediatric dysphagia: a review. JAMA Otolaryngol Head Neck Surg 2020;146(2):183–91.
4. Javia L, Dunham B, Jacobs I. Chapter 90 congenital malformations of the trachea and bronchi. In: Bluestone and stool's pediatric otolaryngology. Fifth Edition. People's Medical Publishing House; 2014. p. 1533–44.
5. Shah RK, Mora BN, Bacha E, et al. The presentation and management of vascular rings: an otolaryngology perspective. Int J Pediatr Otorhinolaryngol 2007;71(1): 57–62.
6. Nelson JS, Hurtado CG, Wearden PD. Surgery for dysphagia lusoria in children. Ann Thorac Surg 2020;109(2):e131–3.
7. Bowder AN, Bence CM, Rymeski BA, et al. Acid suppression duration does not alter anastomotic stricture rates after esophageal atresia with distal tracheoesophageal fistula repair: A prospective multi-institutional cohort study. J Pediatr Surg 2022;57(6):975–80.
8. Patterson KN, Beyene TJ, Gil LA, et al. Procedural and surgical interventions for esophageal stricture secondary to caustic ingestion in children. J Pediatr Surg 2023;58(9):1631–9.
9. Colman K, Simons J, Alper C. Chapter 79 caustic injuries and acquired strictures of the esophagus. In: Bluestone and stool's pediatric otolaryngology. Fifth Edition. People's Medical Publishing House; 2014. p. 1365–80.
10. Davidson JR, McCluney S, Reddy K, et al. Pediatric esophageal dilatations: a cross-specialty experience. J Laparoendosc Adv Surg Tech 2020;30(2):206–9.

Neurogenic Dysphagia

Swapna K. Chandran, MD*, Manon Doucet, MD

KEYWORDS

- Neurogenic dysphagia • Stroke • Parkinson's disease • ALS • MS

KEY POINTS

- Neurogenic dsyphagia needs immediate evaluation for the safety and efficacy of swallowing.
- Various methods of evaluation are utilized and no standard screening exists.
- Various treatment methods involve compensation and/or rehabilitation and have varied results but early intervention leads to the most improvement.

Neurogenic dysphagia is described as dysphagia or dysfunction of the swallowing mechanism in those patients who have suffered neurologic insult or disease. Such diseases include stroke, Parkinson's disease (PD), amyotrophic lateral sclerosis (ALS), and multiple sclerosis (MS), among other neurodegenerative disease processes. Swallowing is a sensorimotor function encompassing about 50 pairs of striated muscles of the upper aerodigestive tract and is a complex interaction of sequential events involving the oral cavity, oropharyngeal structures, and the esophagus. Any neurologic impairment of these structures can cause significant aspiration risk as well as potential malnutrition.

Swallowing is initiated in the forebrain, in the anterior insular cortex and the frontoparietal operculum, including the inferior part of the sensorimotor cortex and part of the premotor cortex. The corticobulbar connections originate in these areas and project to the ipsilateral and the contralateral brainstem nuclei of the main cranial nerves involved in swallowing. The "central pattern originator" for swallowing is located in the medulla oblongata, corresponding to the nucleus tractus solitarius (NTS). The NTS receives afferent input from the nucleus ambiguous, which in turn send efferent fibers to the most important muscles for swallowing.[1,2] The NTS receives its inputs from the oral, pharyngeal, and laryngeal mucosa and can modulate swallowing depend on the bolus properties such as size, texture, and temperature. The 2 areas of the central pattern originators are synchronized to coordinate the bilateral contraction of bilateral muscles of the oropharynx[1] (**Fig. 1**).

Department of Otolaryngology, Head and Neck Surgery and Communicative Disorders, University of Louisville, 529 South Jackson Street, Louisville, KY 40202, USA
* Corresponding author.
E-mail address: Swapna.chandran@louisville.edu

Otolaryngol Clin N Am 57 (2024) 589–597
https://doi.org/10.1016/j.otc.2024.02.023
0030-6665/24/© 2024 Elsevier Inc. All rights reserved.

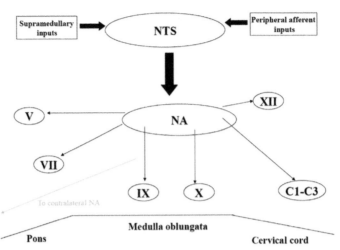

Fig. 1. The figure shows the central program generator (CPG) located in the medulla oblongata and corresponding to the nucleus tractus solitarius (NTS), which receive both ascending and descending inputs and project to the ipsilateral brainstem nucleus such as nucleus ambiguous (NA); nucleus of V, VII, IX, X, and XII cranial nerves; and C1 to C3 tract of the cervical medulla. The existence of 2 CPGs can explain the recovery of the swallowing function after lesion of 1 CPG. (*From* Panebianco M, Marchese-Ragona R, Masiero S, Restivo DA. Dysphagia in neurological diseases: a literature review. Neurol Sci 2020;41(11):3067-73 https://doi.org/10.1007/s10072-020-04495-2 [published Online First: 20200607].)

The following article will outline some of the features of dysphagia and rehabilitative methods for various conditions categorized as neurogenic dysphagia. It can be noted, however, that though there may be different neurologic disease processes that result in dysphagia from impairment from central to peripheral pathways, it is often similar in presentation with impairments in the oral and/or pharyngeal phases, with less likely esophageal phase dysphagia. Rehabilitative efforts are often targeted to achieve safe swallow. A correct and early diagnosis is essential in optimizing outcomes and could be most useful in successful improvement.

STROKE
Diagnosis and Evaluation

Stroke-related dysphagia was previously thought to occur only following brainstem or bilateral cortical strokes, but the development of brain imaging and dynamic swallowing studies have revealed even small, unilateral supratentorial strokes can produce dysphagia.[3] According to the American Stroke Association, stroke is the leading cause of dysphagia, with 25% to 81% experiencing swallow dysfunction within the first 3 days.[3–6] Though the majority of patients have improvement within the first 2 weeks, the American Stroke Association, the American Speech and Language Association, and the Veteran's Health Administration recommend screening for dysphagia and aspiration risk early in patients with stroke prior to oral intake of food and medications.[7,8] Clinical predictors of dysphagia and aspiration include poor nutrition, tube feeding on admission, poor tongue and cough strength, poor secretion management, and the presence of dysphonia, including wet voice and spontaneous cough after swallow. Additionally, lingual function and facial asymmetry are also associated with higher risk of aspiration.[9,10] Varied sources have also noted older age, malnutrition/lower body mass index, subcortical versus cortical involvement, brainstem involvement, corticobulbar tract involvement, white matter involvement, male sex, higher Glasgow Coma Scale, hemorrhagic versus ischemic stroke, anterior or middle cerebral artery involvement, facial palsy, large versus small vessel occlusion, and facial palsy have increased risk.[10] Some studies have also noted intubation, intensive unit stay, and tracheostomy to be independent risks for dysphagia as well.[11] In addition to the physical sequelae from post-stroke dysphagia, it has been also demonstrated that this population are more likely to suffer from post-stroke depression as compared to the general stroke population.[12]

Early identification with a screening tool has been attempted by many researchers, but no validated tool has yet been endorsed. However, the acute stroke dysphagia screening and the Mann Assessment of Swallowing Ability (MASA) are available.[13,14] The MASA is typically administered by speech-language pathologists and is a clinical bedside evaluation that has been validated against the videofluoroscopic swallow study (VFSS). It provides a clear operational definition of dysphagia and aspiration risk.[3,10]

There are 2 levels of evaluation of post-stroke dysphagia: clinical screening evaluation and instrumental examination, which includes functional endoscopic evaluation of swallowing (FEES)and VFSS/modified barium swallow study. It is recommended that all stroke patients have evaluation for risk of dysphagia and/or aspiration.[10] A bedside screening evaluation is designed to be quickly and rapidly administered by health care providers, including speech-language pathologists and trained nursing. There are currently 5 validated screening tools for stroke, yet it has not been determined which is a universal screening tool.[3] In addition to assessment of swallowing safety, cognition, communication, and overall appearance are also evaluated as part of the screening process. Information regarding these deficits aids in the assessment of independence in feeding and oral hygiene which can also be risk factors for pneumonia.

The cranial nerve examination can highlight decreased sensation, range of motion, symmetry, and strength of orofacial musculature that may result in deficits in the oral phase of swallowing. Subjective judgment as well as objective scales such as the Iowa oral pressure instrument (IOPI Medical, Woodinville, WA, USA) for tongue strength and volitional cough strength are also helpful to determine potential deficits in swallowing.[15]

Assessment of swallowing during the clinical screening examination (CSE) can be done at the bedside with multiple trials of each consistency as long as the patient is alert enough to participate. Thin liquids, semisolids, and solid foods are utilized and should begin with small amounts of thin liquid to limit the amount of aspiration should it occur. The volume should increase in gradual, regulated amounts. The same method should be used for semisolids with evaluation of patient-regulated volumes and sequential swallows. The oral cavity should be inspected for residue following ingestion of semisolid and solid foods. The larynx should also be palpated to evaluate the initiation of pharyngeal swallow and laryngeal elevation.

After the clinical evaluation at the bedside, it can be determined if an instrumental assessment of swallowing should be undertaken. In almost every case after stroke, an instrumental examination should be recommended after the CSE.[10] The goals of the instrumental evaluation are evaluation of biomechanical and physiologic function, determination of swallowing safety and efficiency, identification of effective compensatory strategies and rehabilitation approaches, and determination of a safe diet. VFSS was historically the preferred method of evaluation in some instances, especially in stroke, as it allows for the direct assessment of oral, pharyngeal, and esophageal phases, which helps with development of a rehabilitative plan. The specific areas of impairment can be seen through all the swallowing phases, such as differences in hyoid excursion, laryngeal elevation, tongue base retraction, pharyngeal shortening, and timing of bolus movement. FEES, which incorporates a videoendoscopic approach to evaluation, is also utilized, especially in rehabilitative facilities and in cases of medical fragility. In the last few decades, it has been established as an equivalent method of evaluation.[16] FEES can also be used to serially assess the patient for signs of improvement without exposing the patient to radiation. Similar feeding protocols are used for the instrumental assessment as the CSE, and careful attention to particular deficits from the stroke outside of swallow, such as cognitive and inhibition deficits or limb paralysis, should be accounted for during the administration of the food bolus. Knowledge of the cognitive impairment will also help determine the types of compensatory strategies the patient is able to self-employ.

Management

Traditional strategies for treatment of post-stroke dysphagia include compensatory mechanisms and rehabilitative options, which are often individualized based on the comprehensive evaluation. Within the rehabilitative options, neurostimulation and biofeedback have been utilized to enhance recovery potential.[5] Compensatory strategies offer alteration of diet consistencies and postural techniques such as chin tuck position and swallow strategies.[17] Rehabilitative methods include swallowing exercises such as tongue exercises, effortful swallow, and Mendelsohn's maneuver and the Shaker exercise.[18,19] Other techniques of rehabilitation have included strategies to promote recovery through enhancing neural plasticity and utilizing central, peripheral, and sensory stimulation. Neural plasticity can be promoted by noninvasive brain stimulation[20] (repetitive transcranial direct stimulation to modulate brain activity to induce long-lasting change in synaptic plasticity).[21] Stimulation of the peripheral pathway is achieved with pharyngeal electrical stimulation which offers direct stimulation of the pharyngeal mucosa through an intraluminal catheter. As with most therapeutic methods, success in swallowing improvement is most likely in the first 2 weeks after acute stroke.[5]

It should be noted that when considering a gastrostomy tube (G tube) for dysphagia after stroke, it may be beneficial to attain improved nutritional status. However, studies have not demonstrated an increased survival after placement of the G tube.[8]

Surgical interventions usually are aimed at targeting the upper esophageal sphincter (UES) to better allow passage of the bolus. Interventions such as botulinum toxin injection, dilation, and myotomy improve the passage of the bolus into the esophagus, but efficacy can be best determined by findings on instrumental assessments.

PARKINSON'S DISEASE
Evaluation and Diagnosis

PD is 1 of the most common neurologic disorders and the second most common cause of neurogenic dysphagia.[22] PD primarily involves degeneration of the nigrostriatal dopaminergic pathway, and it also impacts other neural systems, including bulbar functions such as speech and swallowing. As in stroke, dysphagia often results in aspiration, pneumonia, and malnutrition. Dysphagia has a prevalence between 11% and 87% depending on the severity of the disease.[23] Impairments in all the phases of swallowing are possible, yet in contrast to stroke, esophageal motility is more common and evaluation with instrumental assessments such as VFSS and FEES is essential. Esophageal manometry can also be helpful to assess passage of food through the esophagus. The use manometry has demonstrated that differences in the pharyngeal contraction and upper esophageal opening relate to stage of disease and can help determine treatment options.[24] Many of the strategies utilized for assessment in stroke can be translated to PD patients, with special note of other impairments such as posture and cognition that may limit the patient's ability to cooperate with assessment and rehabilitative strategies.

Management

Dopamine agonist medications are the gold standard used in the treatment of PD, though have inconsistent results when looking at dysphagia—with some improvement in bolus formation, transit time, and residue in the pharynx.[23,25] Treatment strategies utilized in stroke patients such as traditional swallowing exercises and neurostimulation have a role in rehabilitation as well, with variable results.[24] Likewise, neurostimulation interventions such as deep brain stimulation has also had inconsistent results in swallowing function and aspiration.[25] A combination of treatment modalities, such as deep brain stimulation and biofeedback, lead to improvements in swallowing timing and latency but little effect on swallowing safety. Thus, the overall efficacy is still debated.[23]

AMYOTROPHIC LATERAL SCLEROSIS

ALS is a neurologic disorder involving both the upper and lower motor neurons. A large percentage of patients with ALS experience bulbar dysfunction, resulting in dysphagia.[26] Several studies estimate approximately 85% of ALS patients have dysphagia.[27–29] In approximately 30% of patients, these bulbar symptoms including dysarthria and dysphagia present prior to the symptoms involving the spinal system.[30] Of ALS patients who first present with only 1 functional impairment, dysphagia was 4 times more likely to occur as the first impairment.[31] As such, these patients may first present to the otolaryngologist, prior to a diagnosis of ALS by the neurologist.

Patients can present with difficulty swallowing, but their complaints may be more subtle, such as unintentional weight loss, coughing of choking with eating, length of time needed to eat, or difficulty with saliva management.[26] Symptoms are often accompanied by dysarthria. A common finding is weakness of the tongue musculature, which is disproportionately weak in ALS.[30] VFSS and FEES should be performed early as in other neurologic disorders; however, electromyography of submental, laryngeal, pharyngeal, or diaphragmatic sensors or a sequential water swallowing test should be evaluated. VFSS was found to be the most sensitive in detecting early changes in swallowing.[32] The oral phase of swallowing is most commonly affected.

As ALS is a fatal disease with no cure, treatment primarily relates to symptom management. Unfortunately, decreased tongue strength at time of diagnosis has been shown to be associated with a decreased survival time.[33] Most individuals with ALS die on an average of 2 to 4 years from symptom onset, and bronchopneumonia followed by aspiration pneumonia is the leading cause of death.[34] Speech and swallowing therapy plays an important role. Weight loss and inadequate nutrition can accelerate progression of the disease; therefore, timing of G tube placement is an important consideration. Though results are mixed, studies showed a longer survival in ALS patients with G tube compared to those without it.[35]

MULTIPLE SCLEROSIS

MS is an autoimmune disease with a predilection for young adults, specifically young females. The disease is defined by relapsing-remitting attacks of inflammation, demyelination, and axonal damage in the central nervous system, leading to various degrees and spectra of neurologic symptoms and disability.[36] These symptoms tend to worsen over the patient's lifetime, but due to the relapsing-remitting nature, it can be challenging to diagnose and treat.

The role of dysphagia in MS has been described as early as the nineteenth century.[37] MS can affect the process of swallowing at any of the 4 stages of swallowing secondary to MS lesions affecting the corticobulbar tract, cranial nerves, the cerebellum, and the brainstem. Many studies have established that dysphagia occurs more frequently in the MS population than the general population. In a meta-analysis conducted by Mirmosayyeb and colleagues,[37] it was concluded that the prevalence of dysphagia in MS patients is approximately 45%.

Diagnosis of dysphagia in the patient with MS can be challenging, as symptoms can be intermittent and difficult to categorize. However, early diagnosis can prevent complications such as aspiration pneumonia, weight loss, and airway obstruction, underlying the importance of regular screening. Several screening tools have been developed, most notably the Dysphagia in Multiple Sclerosis Questionnaire (DYMUS) and the MASA, although many are used.[10,38,39] The DYMUS is a validated questionnaire with 10 questions.[40] In summary, there are many approaches to screen for dysphagia, and further assessment can be performed with instrumental tools such as VFSS and FEES.

Treatment options are limited and the effectiveness of treatment has not been well described. Neuromuscular electrostimulation applied slightly above the patient's UES and stimulation of the vagal nerve through implantation have demonstrated variable results but showed some promise.[41]

SUMMARY

Neurogenic dysphagia encompasses a host of neurologic conditions, but the overall assessment with clinical and instrumental tools is paramount to the accurate determination of swallowing safety and an appropriate diet. Compensatory and rehabilitative methods are also fairly similar in these conditions but should be individualized to patients based on the comprehensive, multidisciplinary assessment. Variable results are expected, but the consensus seems to be that early intervention has the most potential for improvement in dysphagia.

CLINICS CARE POINTS

- Swallowing is a sensorimotor function encompassing about 50 pairs of striated muscles of the upper aerodigestive tract and is a complex interaction of sequential events involving the oral cavity, oropharyngeal structures, and the esophagus.
- Any neurologic impairment of these structures can cause neurogenic dysphagia.
- It is recommended that all stroke patients receive a comprehensive dysphagia assessment as studies reveal even small strokes can result in dysphagia.
- Clinical screening evaluations and instrumental examinations such as FEES and VFSS are recommended basic tools for assessing dysphagia in stroke, Parkinson's, ALS, and MS patients.
- Treatment options are limited to therapeutic interventions/maneuvers and neuroelectrical stimulation and should be employed as early as possible.
- Some treatments have incorporated deep brain stimulators to help control tremor and improve dysphagia.

- G-tube placement has not been shown to increase survival in populations other than ALS patients.

REFERENCES

1. Panebianco M, Marchese-Ragona R, Masiero S, et al. Dysphagia in neurological diseases: a literature review. Neurol Sci 2020;41(11):3067–73.
2. Jean A. Brain stem control of swallowing: neuronal network and cellular mechanisms. Physiol Rev 2001;81(2):929–69.
3. Felix CC, Joseph ME, Daniels SK. Clinical Decision Making in Patients with Stroke-Related Dysphagia. Semin Speech Lang 2019;40(3):188–202.
4. Behera A, Read D, Jackson N, et al. A Validated Swallow Screener for Dysphagia and Aspiration in Patients with Stroke. J Stroke Cerebrovasc Dis 2018;27(7): 1897–904.
5. Cheng I, Sasegbon A, Hamdy S. Effects of Neurostimulation on Poststroke Dysphagia: A Synthesis of Current Evidence From Randomized Controlled Trials. Neuromodulation 2021;24(8):1388–401.
6. Chen S, Xian W, Cheng S, et al. Risk of regurgitation and aspiration in patients infused with different volumes of enteral nutrition. Asia Pac J Clin Nutr 2015; 24(2):212–8.
7. Sreedharan SE, Sayed JV, Vipina VP, et al. Dysphagia Continues to Impact Recovery at One Year After Stroke-An Observational Study. J Stroke Cerebrovasc Dis 2022;31(8):106545.
8. Patita M, Nunes G, Grunho M, et al. Endoscopic gastrostomy for nutritional support in post-stroke dysphagia. Nutr Hosp 2021;38(6):1126–31.
9. Rosenbek JC, McCullough GH, Wertz RT. Is the information about a test important? Applying the methods of evidence-based medicine to the clinical examination of swallowing. J Commun Disord 2004;37(5):437–50.
10. Jones CA, Colletti CM, Ding MC. Post-stroke Dysphagia: Recent Insights and Unanswered Questions. Curr Neurol Neurosci Rep 2020;20(12):61.
11. Dunn K, Rumbach A. Incidence and Risk Factors for Dysphagia Following Nontraumatic Subarachnoid Hemorrhage: A Retrospective Cohort Study. Dysphagia 2019;34(2):229–39.
12. Horn J, Simpson KN, Simpson AN, et al. Incidence of Poststroke Depression in Patients With Poststroke Dysphagia. Am J Speech Lang Pathol 2022;31(4): 1836–44.
13. Antonios N, Carnaby-Mann G, Crary M, et al. Analysis of a physician tool for evaluating dysphagia on an inpatient stroke unit: the modified Mann Assessment of Swallowing Ability. J Stroke Cerebrovasc Dis 2010;19(1):49–57.
14. Edmiaston J, Connor LT, Loehr L, et al. Validation of a dysphagia screening tool in acute stroke patients. Am J Crit Care 2010;19(4):357–64.
15. Edmiaston J, Connor LT, Steger-May K, et al. A simple bedside stroke dysphagia screen, validated against videofluoroscopy, detects dysphagia and aspiration with high sensitivity. J Stroke Cerebrovasc Dis 2014;23(4):712–6.
16. Labeit B, Ahring S, Boehmer M, et al. Comparison of Simultaneous Swallowing Endoscopy and Videofluoroscopy in Neurogenic Dysphagia. J Am Med Dir Assoc 2022;23(8):1360–6.
17. Bath PM, Lee HS, Everton LF. Swallowing therapy for dysphagia in acute and subacute stroke. Cochrane Database Syst Rev 2018;10(10):CD000323.

18. Mendelsohn MS, McConnel FM. Function in the pharyngoesophageal segment. Laryngoscope 1987;97(4):483–9.

19. Shaker R, Easterling C, Kern M, et al. Rehabilitation of swallowing by exercise in tube-fed patients with pharyngeal dysphagia secondary to abnormal UES opening. Gastroenterology 2002;122(5):1314–21.

20. Lamola G, Fanciullacci C, Rossi B, et al. Clinical evidences of brain plasticity in stroke patients. Arch Ital Biol 2014;152(4):259–71.

21. Hallett M, Epstein CM, Berardelli A, et al. Topics in transcranial magnetic stimulation. Suppl Clin neurophysiol 2000;53:301–11.

22. Takizawa C, Gemmell E, Kenworthy J, et al. A Systematic Review of the Prevalence of Oropharyngeal Dysphagia in Stroke, Parkinson's Disease, Alzheimer's Disease, Head Injury, and Pneumonia. Dysphagia 2016;31(3):434–41.

23. Lechien JR, Saussez S, Schindler A, et al. Clinical outcomes of laryngopharyngeal reflux treatment: A systematic review and meta-analysis. Laryngoscope 2019; 129(5):1174–87.

24. Cosentino G, Todisco M, Giudice C, et al. Assessment and treatment of neurogenic dysphagia in stroke and Parkinson's disease. Curr Opin Neurol 2022; 35(6):741–52.

25. Gandhi P, Steele CM. Effectiveness of Interventions for Dysphagia in Parkinson Disease: A Systematic Review. Am J Speech Lang Pathol 2022;31(1):463–85.

26. Lee J, Madhavan A, Krajewski E, et al. Assessment of dysarthria and dysphagia in patients with amyotrophic lateral sclerosis: Review of the current evidence. Muscle Nerve 2021;64(5):520–31.

27. Chen A, Garrett CG. Otolaryngologic presentations of amyotrophic lateralsclerosis. Otolaryngol Head Neck Surg 2005;132(3):500–4.

28. Ruoppolo G, Schettino I, Frasca V, et al. Dysphagia in amyotrophic lateral sclerosis: prevalence and clinical findings. Acta Neurol Scand 2013;128(6):397–401.

29. Wang BJ, Carter FL, Altman KW. Relationship between Dysarthria and Oral-Oropharyngeal Dysphagia: The present evidence. Ear Nose Throat J 2020. https://doi.org/10.1177/0145561320951647. 145561320951647.

30. Haverkamp LJ, Appel V, Appel SH. Natural history of amyotrophic lateral sclerosis in a database population. Validation of a scoring system and a model for survival prediction. Brain 1995;118(Pt 3):707–19.

31. Robison R, DiBiase L, Ashley A, et al. Swallowing Safety and Efficiency Impairment Profiles in Individuals with Amyotrophic Lateral Sclerosis. Dysphagia 2022;37(3):644–54.

32. Briani C, Marcon M, Ermani M, et al. Radiological evidence of subclinical dysphagia in motor neuron disease. J Neurol 1998;245(4):211–6.

33. Weikamp JG, Schelhaas HJ, Hendriks JC, et al. Prognostic value of decreased tongue strength on survival time in patients with amyotrophic lateral sclerosis. J Neurol 2012;259(11):2360–5.

34. Burkhardt C, Neuwirth C, Sommacal A, et al. Is survival improved by the use of NIV and PEG in amyotrophic lateral sclerosis (ALS)? A post-mortem study of 80 ALS patients. PLoS One 2017;12(5):e0177555.

35. Sulistyo A, Abrahao A, Freitas ME, et al. Enteral tube feeding for amyotrophic lateral sclerosis/motor neuron disease. Cochrane Database Syst Rev 2023;8(8): CD004030.

36. Harbo HF, Gold R, Tintoré M. Sex and gender issues in multiple sclerosis. Ther Adv Neurol Disord 2013;6(4):237–48.

37. Mirmosayyeb O, Ebrahimi N, Shekarian A, et al. Prevalence of dysphagia in patients with multiple sclerosis: A systematic review and meta-analysis. J Clin Neurosci 2023;108:84–94.
38. Ansari NN, Tarameshlu M, Ghelichi L. Dysphagia In Multiple Sclerosis Patients: Diagnostic And Evaluation Strategies. Degener Neurol Neuromuscul Dis 2020; 10:15–28.
39. Mann G. MASA, the Mann assessment of swallowing ability. Florence, KY: Singular Thomson Learning; 2002.
40. Bergamaschi R, Crivelli P, Rezzani C, et al. The DYMUS questionnaire for the assessment of dysphagia in multiple sclerosis. J Neurol Sci 2008;269(1–2): 49–53.
41. Alali D, Ballard K, Vucic S, et al. Dysphagia in Multiple Sclerosis: Evaluation and Validation of the DYMUS Questionnaire. Dysphagia 2018;33(3):273–81.

Neurologic Dysphagia

Jillian Nyswonger Sugg, MS, CCC-SLP[a], Janet Waimin Lee, MD[b],*

KEYWORDS

- Dysphagia • Pediatric • Neurologic • Cerebral palsy • Prematurity
- Traumatic brain injury

KEY POINTS

- Patients with neurologic/neuromuscular disorders often have multiple contributors to dysphagia.
- There is a wide range of symptoms and severity that can be seen in patients with neurologic dysphagia, so feeding/swallowing therapy strategies should be individualized.
- Shared decision-making and clear communication are critical in caring for patients with evolving neurologic disorders.

INTRODUCTION

Neurologic/neuromuscular causes of dysphagia include cerebral palsy (CP), seizure disorders, hydrocephalus, congenital brain malformations, traumatic brain injury (TBI), tumors, genetic abnormalities, and muscular dystrophies. Dysphagia in the neurologic pediatric population varies significantly in severity, domains of swallowing impacted, and prognosis. Many individuals with neurologic dysphagia present with reduced strength and coordination of oral, pharyngeal, and esophageal swallowing function, which can lead to poor nutrition, impaired growth, and increased risk of aspiration and associated respiratory issues. Impaired laryngeal sensation is also common in this population due to neurologic etiology and/or other medical comorbidity such as gastroesophageal reflux disease/laryngopharyngeal reflux, leading to an increased risk of silent aspiration.[1,2] As advances in the care of medically complex and extremely premature infants have been made, survival of children with neurologic and neuromuscular disorders has improved, making the early identification and appropriate management of their dysphagia increasingly important.

Differentiation between causes of dysphagia in medically complex children can be especially difficult, as these patients frequently have multiple comorbidities that may affect their sensory processing and behavior in addition to their strictly neurologic

[a] Department of Head and Neck Surgery & Communication Sciences, Division of Speech Pathology and Audiology, Duke University, DUMC 3887, Durham, NC 27710, USA; [b] Department of Head and Neck Surgery & Communication Sciences, Division of Pediatric Otolaryngology, Duke University, DUMC 3805, Durham, NC 27710, USA
* Corresponding author.
E-mail address: janet.w.lee@duke.edu

Otolaryngol Clin N Am 57 (2024) 599–608
https://doi.org/10.1016/j.otc.2024.03.005
0030-6665/24/© 2024 Elsevier Inc. All rights reserved.

and neuromuscular function. For the purpose of this review, we will refer to disorders, which affect the central nervous system and musculature as "neurologic" or "neuromuscular," while we will refer to neuropsychiatric and behavioral concerns that may affect oral intake such as autism spectrum disorder, textural aversions, and "picky" eating as "behavioral."[3] Children with autism spectrum disorder often present with feeding difficulties that are considered behavioral/sensory in nature resulting in food refusals, texture aversions, and/or strong feeding preferences with no medical or physiologic explanation.[4] Behavioral feeding difficulties may co-occur alongside oropharyngeal skill deficits/dysphagia but often present without identifiable physiologic deficits in oral motor or pharyngeal function.[3,4] For this review, we will focus on clinical presentation and considerations for the management of neurologically based true oral/pharyngeal dysphagia. For further discussion of behavioral/sensory-based feeding difficulties such as those seen in children with autism spectrum disorder, please refer to the excellent reviews available throughout the literature.[4,5]

ETIOLOGIES OF NEUROLOGIC/NEUROMUSCULAR DYSPHAGIA
Infants with Neurologic Insult

Infants with history of neurologic insult due to pre/perinatal complications including hypoxic ischemic encephalopathy, neonatal stroke, intraventricular hemorrhage (IVH), periventricular leukomalacia (PVL), and their sequelae (such as seizures) often present with dysphagia and feeding difficulties. Severity and clinical presentation of these difficulties varies significantly depending on the area of neurologic damage, comorbidities, and gestational/chronologic age.

Clinical presentation of dysphagia during the neonatal/early infancy period may include poor behavioral state regulation, poor alertness, oral motor dysfunction and disorganization, poor endurance leading to early onset of fatigue with associated deterioration of skills/coordination, increased tone, sucking problems, swallowing problems, and aspiration.[6] Specific characteristics observed in many of these patients include impaired secretion management, pooling in the oral cavity, loss of liquid from the lips, reduced rooting and shallow latch during breastfeeding, extended feeding durations, falling asleep during feeding attempts, coughing, gagging, vomiting, nasopharyngeal reflux, regurgitation, breath-holding or respiratory issues associated with poor suck-swallow-breathe coordination, increased work of breathing (at times indicated by nasal flaring), poor swallow initiation, absent cough reflex, and aspiration.[6–8] These deficits can lead to poor growth/weight gain, need for nonoral nutrition/hydration, increased risk of aspiration/associated respiratory issues, and long-term feeding difficulties/dysphagia. Feeding difficulties in this population contributes to an extended length of hospitalization.[7] These deficits present during both breastfeeding and bottle-feeding attempts; therefore, all infants with neurologic involvement of this nature should receive feeding support, regardless of the method of feeding.[7,8] Prolonged dysphagia and feeding difficulties, particularly associated with neurologic injuries related to extreme prematurity and injuries to the brainstem, frequently present with more severe dysphagia and require long-term tube feeding.[7–9]

Cerebral Palsy

Children with a history of neurologic insult in infancy (specifically IVH, PVL, and neonatal stroke) are at an increased risk of later diagnosis of CP. The majority of children with CP present with oropharyngeal dysphagia and/or feeding difficulties.[10] Presentation and severity of dysphagia in this population varies, with an increased risk of more severe dysphagia associated with more severe motor impairments.[10,11]

Many children with CP demonstrate dysphagia across the oral and pharyngeal phases of swallowing due to reduced control/coordination of swallowing function.[10,12,13] Specific characteristics of dysphagia in children with CP include sialorrhea, reduced lip closure, reduced lingual control/coordination, prolonged tongue thrust pattern, exaggerated bite reflex, delayed posterior bolus transfer, oral hypersensitivity, anterior loss of liquids/food, slow eating/extended mealtime durations, coughing during oral feeding, texture selectivity/slow progression of oral diet, and nasopharyngeal reflux.[11,12,14] The impaired timing and coordination of pharyngeal swallowing and laryngeal closure resulting in more difficulties swallowing liquids than solids.[11] Instrumental assessments in this population reveal specific pharyngeal phase deficits including delayed swallow initiation with posterior spillage of bolus prior to pharyngeal swallow trigger, piecemeal swallowing, incomplete tongue base retraction/reduced pharyngeal propulsion leading to pharyngeal residue, and reduced laryngeal closure/sensation leading to silent aspiration.[11,12] Esophageal phase deficits may occur in this population; however, these deficits are often related to comorbid issues such as scoliosis/kyphosis and gastrointestinal system involvement.

Assessment and intervention of dysphagia and feeding difficulties in this population should be patient-centered and individualized based on patient needs, family and patient goals, overall medical status, and specific clinical presentation. Given the increased risk of pharyngeal phase deficits and silent aspiration, instrumental swallowing assessment are indicated, especially in younger patients and those with more severe motor impairments, as the risk of aspiration usually decreases with age and neurodevelopmental progress.[11–13] However, some children with CP demonstrated increased symptoms of dysphagia upon onset of puberty due to increased nutritional needs and/or worsening of scoliosis/kyphosis.[11] Full oral feeding may not be a realistic goal for some children with CP.[11] Feeding/swallowing therapy for this population is essential and may include strategies to optimize positioning, improve oral sensorimotor function, identify and implement compensatory techniques and aspiration precautions, provide caregiver training/education, update oral diet recommendations, and coordinate/collaborate with the medical team.

Dysphagia in Children with Acquired Neurologic Damage

Dysphagia in the pediatric population after TBI is associated with physiologic and cognitive deficits that impact not only oral/pharyngeal swallowing function but also feeding behaviors. Incidence of dysphagia varies across age and population but has been reported to be fairly low (<10%); however, increased severity of TBI and prolonged intubation/ventilation have been associated with a higher risk of dysphagia in children with a history of TBI.[15] Specific characteristics of dysphagia include oral motor deficits, atypical tongue reflexes, reduced jaw stability, reduced bolus control, delayed posterior bolus propulsion, impaired mastication with slow/effortful chewing, reduced lip closure, piecemeal swallowing, absent/delayed initiation of swallowing, reduced oral/pharyngeal sensation, reduced laryngeal elevation, and reduced/impaired strength, tone, and range of motion of oral/pharyngeal musculature.[16] Cognitive issues may result in feeding difficulties due to atypical feeding behaviors including difficulty with initiation of oral motor movements such as mouth opening, increased impulsivity and reduced attention during oral feeding, and reduced awareness of deficits.[16]

Children with dysphagia related to brain tumors and/or complications of their treatment (such as posterior fossa tumor resection or radiation) can have variable presentations. Symptoms vary based on location and size of tumors and may change over time depending on specific diagnosis and treatment methods. As the posterior fossa region is the most common site of childhood brain tumors and the structures/lower cranial nerves within this area are critical for neurologic control of swallowing, these tumors and their resection frequently result in immediate postoperative dysphagia. Dysphagia after posterior fossa tumor resection may present with severe loss of swallowing function, delayed-absent swallow initiation, reduced laryngeal closure, reduced laryngeal sensation, aspiration of oral intake with or without sensory response, reduced bolus control, impaired chewing skills, and/or sialorrhea and difficulty with secretion management.[17,18] Postoperative recovery of swallow function is highly variable across patients and may occur up to months after surgical intervention; however, slow progress in swallowing function initially after surgery may indicate an increased risk of need for nonoral means of nutrition/hydration (ie, via g-tube) during rehabilitation. Use of instrumental swallowing assessment methods may be warranted for this population, especially for children who experience a more difficult postoperative course with increased swallowing difficulties/aspiration. Many children experience long-term feeding difficulties after treatment of brain tumors due to numerous factors including swallowing deficits, lack of age-appropriate feeding experiences, and refusal behaviors.[17]

In children with seizure disorders/epilepsy, the effects of medication or medication changes, potential for ongoing seizures resulting in further neurologic damage, comorbid issues/medical complexity, and overall medical/neurodevelopmental prognosis should be considered in the management of dysphagia and feeding difficulties. Deficits may include reduced alertness/reduced behavioral feeding readiness, atypical oral reflexes, difficulty with initiating volitional oral motor movements, slowed/effortful movements, oral sensorimotor dysfunction, poor bolus control, sialorrhea and reduced secretion management, pooling and anterior loss of liquids, slow-absent posterior bolus transit, reduced-absent swallow initiation, and/or reduced laryngeal closure/sensation. All of these factors can increase the risks of inadequate nutrition/hydration via oral feeding alone as well as the risk of aspiration, so nonoral means to optimize nutrition/hydration may be necessary. Treatment of seizures may also impact feeding and swallowing with some medications increasing somnolence and reducing patients' ability to participate in oral feeding/feeding and swallowing therapy.

Progressive Neuromuscular Disease

Pediatric patients with progressive neuromuscular diseases including myotonic dystrophy, Duchenne muscular dystrophy, spinal muscular atrophy, and Pompe disease frequently experience dysphagia that varies in specific deficits, severity, and functional impact across diagnoses and age groups. Dysphagia is a frequent symptom of neuromuscular diseases, occurring in ~35% to 80% of patients across the life span.[19] In most patients in this population, the oral phase of swallowing is most impaired, followed by pharyngeal phase deficits, and with most deficits associated with muscle weakness and atypical swallowing patterns resulting in more difficulty with solid food consistencies compared to liquids.[13,20–22] Specific deficits may include anterior loss due to reduced lip closure, piecemeal swallowing/multiple swallows per bolus, and/or reduced tongue base retraction/reduced pharyngeal propulsion resulting in pharyngeal residue after the swallow.[13,20,21] With disease progression, the cough reflex may deteriorate, increasing the risk of silent aspiration and resulting respiratory issues, such as aspiration pneumonia, which has a major impact on overall prognosis in this population.[19,22] Assessment and management of feeding difficulties and dysphagia in patients with progressive neuromuscular diseases should consider disease progression and involve close collaboration with medical team and other providers to optimize safety and efficiency of oral intake.

Congenital Neurologic Abnormality

Congenital neurologic abnormalities such as Chiari malformation, myelomeningocele, microcephaly, and hydrocephalus may result in dysphagia, oftentimes, due to increased intracranial pressure and/or brainstem/cranial nerve compression impacting the medullary swallowing center.[23–25]

Infants and children with dysphagia related to brainstem and lower cranial nerve compression may present with symptoms including poor weight gain/failure to thrive, regurgitation of oral intake and secretions, nasopharyngeal regurgitation, prolonged feeding durations, coughing during oral feedings, impaired posterior bolus propulsion, reduced volume of oral intake, aspiration due to impaired laryngeal closure/vocal fold paralysis, impaired upper esophageal sphincter function (cricopharyngeal achalasia), pharyngeal and esophageal dysmotility, and reduced sensation of the pharynx/airway.[25,26] More severe vagal nerve compression, as seen in those with Chiari malformation types II and III, may result in more severe dysphagia related to decreased laryngeal tone, laryngomalacia, vocal fold paralysis, stridor, impaired voicing, aspiration during oral intake, and airway obstruction that can lead to need for tracheostomy.

Dysphagia in this population is typically progressive and may present before more severe symptoms of brainstem dysfunction.[26,27] Infants typically present with more rapid deterioration of swallowing function, while older children and adults typically demonstrate more gradual progression. Surgical intervention to decompress the brainstem prior to onset of other, more severe symptoms of brainstem dysfunction often results in improvement in swallowing function, with mild cases improving rapidly and more severe cases demonstrating slower, less profound improvements.[26,28,29]

Genetic Syndromes Impacting Neurologic Status

Dysphagia in pediatric patients with genetic syndromes impacting neurologic status and neurodevelopment is variable. These patients may present with other comorbid diagnoses such as craniofacial anomalies, airway anomalies, immune defects, congenital cardiac disease, gastrointestinal system abnormalities, cognitive impairment, abnormal muscle tone, and/or muscle weakness, all of which can contribute to the severity and complexity of dysphagia and feeding difficulties. Assessment and intervention of feeding difficulties and dysphagia in this population is warranted to optimize oral feeding safety and efficiency in order to reduce aspiration risk, support growth and weight gain, promote positive oral feeding experiences, facilitate improved oral motor function, decrease oral sensory difficulties, and utilize compensatory measures (positioning, utensil modification, thickening of liquids, and so forth) to improve safety/efficiency of oral intake.

One of the most common genetic syndromes associated with dysphagia and feeding difficulties is Trisomy 21 (Down syndrome), with dysfunction related to a combination of hypotonia, impaired neuromotor control, and dental/orofacial differences including relative macroglossia and open-mouth posture.[30] Infants with Trisomy 21 may present with symptoms of oral phase dysphagia including delayed suckling patterns, reduced lip closure, reduced suction generation with a tendency toward compression pattern for the extraction of liquids from the nipple rather than use of negative pressure, tongue thrust, prolonged feeding durations, coughing or choking during oral feeds, noisy breathing during oral feedings, oxygen desaturations/cyanosis during oral feeds, and uncoordinated suck–swallow–breathe pattern.[30–32] Older infants and toddlers with Trisomy 21 may present with oral phase swallowing deficits including oral motor and sensory difficulties, open-mouth posture, drooling, reduced tongue control, impaired mastication, prolonged tongue thrust pattern, and/or choking/gagging with oral intake.

These problems can increase difficulties with transitioning to solids, prolonged feeding/mealtime durations, difficulty maintaining optimal nutrition/hydration via oral feeding alone.[30–32] Many infants and toddlers/children with Trisomy 21 also present with pharyngeal phase deficits including delayed timing of swallow initiation, deep laryngeal penetration, aspiration, nasopharyngeal regurgitation, pharyngeal residue after the swallow, and upper esophageal sphincter dysfunction.[31–33] Aspiration in infants was most often silent in this population.[31–33] Patients with congenital heart disease, laryngomalacia, desaturations during oral feeds, airway/respiratory anomalies, prematurity, and poor weight gain are at an increased risk of aspiration.[32,33] Due to the documented prevalence of pharyngeal dysphagia and aspiration in this population, the most recent American Academy of Pediatrics Health Supervision for Children with Down syndrome provided a recommendation to "refer all infants with marked hypotonia, slow feeding, choking with feeds, recurrent pneumonia, or other recurrent or persistent respiratory symptoms and unexplained failure to thrive for a radiographic swallowing assessment."[34]

SIALORRHEA

In children with dysphagia of neurologic origin, sialorrhea can be a complicating concern. Sialorrhea can be impactful to patient care in many ways, including the social stigma of visible "drooling," difficulties in keeping the child and their clothing clean, dermatitis, and even aspiration pneumonia. In addition to speech and swallowing therapy, the mainstays of medical treatment start with anticholinergic medications. Systemic medications such as glycopyrrolate and scopolamine are very effective in reducing salivary production but can also thicken secretions and cause side effects such as tachycardia, urinary retention, and dry eyes. Glycopyrrolate may require administration up to 3 times daily, which can be cumbersome, but does allow for frequent titration. Scopolamine patches are longer acting but use in smaller children may be challenging as families must understand appropriate use of fractions of patches at home without cutting the patch itself. Topical treatment of the buccal mucosa with atropine can help target minor salivary glands, which produce more of the thicker mucous component of saliva, but this can also be logistically challenging. Treatment with injection of the major salivary glands with botulinum toxin can be very effective and last 3 months or more, but this may require anesthesia in children that are combative with the procedure. Like anticholinergic therapy, treatment with botulinum toxin for sialorrhea can cause thickened secretions.[35] Although the effects of botulinum toxin are not permanent, they cannot be reversed. More durable options for the management of sialorrhea include parotid duct ligation, submandibular gland excision or duct ligation, or salivary gland ablation via sclerotherapy.

GOALS OF CARE

With the progression of neurologic disease, risk of aspiration and likelihood of need for nonoral means nutrition/hydration increases. The focus of treatment in pediatric patients with severe disease progression may shift from promoting safety/efficiency of oral feeding to promoting quality of life via oral feeds for pleasure combined with reliance on nonoral feeding for nutrition/hydration. Shared decision-making and acceptance of potential risks associated with aspiration occurring with oral intake is critical.

Special consideration should also be given to severe brainstem tumors with poor prognosis in children, such as diffuse intrinsic pontine glioma. These are associated with early symptoms of dysphagia including reduced secretion management, increased coughing, and reduced volume of oral intake. With treatment, many of these children make short-term improvements in oral feeding; however, as the disease progresses, swallowing deficits notably increase. In these children, nonoral feeding is frequently utilized to reduce aspiration and optimize nutrition/hydration status while oral intake is limited to small tastes for pleasure/quality of life purposes.[17]

CONSIDERATIONS FOR EVALUATION AND TREATMENT OF NEUROLOGIC PEDIATRIC DYSPHAGIA

Evaluation of swallowing function in infants and children typically includes clinical feeding/swallowing evaluation and may or may not include instrumental swallowing assessment.

Infants and young children, especially those with neurologic system involvement, are at a higher risk of not only aspiration but also silent aspiration related to impaired laryngeal sensation.[3,36–38] Previous studies have shown that children with neurologic dysphagia most often exhibit silent aspiration with thin liquids compared to other consistencies.[39,40] Given this and the frequency of comorbid medical conditions placing them at higher risk for respiratory complications related to aspiration, instrumental swallow assessment tools such as videofluoroscopic swallow study (VFSS) and fiberoptic endoscopic evaluation of swallowing (FEES) should be considered.

Pediatric patients with neurologic system involvement, particularly when severe, often require nonoral means of nutrition/hydration and may have minimal oral feeding experiences.[14] These patients, who are essentially nil per os (NPO), are at high risk of aspiration and often have difficulty consuming sufficient quantities of barium and/or participating enough during VFSS to facilitate successful, meaningful assessment.[1,41,42] Consideration of FEES and/or ongoing close clinical assessment by an experienced speech/language pathologist (SLP)/feeding therapist is warranted.

At times, dysphagia may be compounded by gross motor impairments and/or comorbid musculoskeletal issues that contribute to positioning difficulties. Considering the impact of positioning as well as limitations in optimizing, positioning is an important component of assessment and intervention in this population.

Feeding/swallowing therapy is essential for pediatric patients with dysphagia and underlying neurologic system involvement. However, many of these patients may be unable to travel to larger academic hospitals to receive therapy from specialized providers/multidisciplinary teams. Often, these patients must rely on community providers, which can present problems since many community-based feeding therapists (SLP/occupational therapist [OT]) may not have the same level of experience with treating medically complex patients. Consideration of a collaborative approach between hospital-based SLP/feeding therapists and local providers may improve quality of care, reduce unnecessary/unhelpful instrumental assessments, and ultimately improve the care of complex patients.

Caregiver/parent training and education is also a critical component of feeding therapy for this population. Clear communication between treatment teams and patients' families can help optimize understanding of expectations and foster an ongoing relationship. Because patients with neurologic dysphagia may experience evolution of their prognoses as well as their clinical status over time, open communication and a collaborative approach to care can be important to facilitate increased acceptance of adjustments in feeding recommendations. Ongoing reassessment is warranted as infants/children make progress in their oral feeding skills. This can be completed by an experienced SLP/feeding therapist through ongoing clinical assessment but may also include repeat instrumental swallow assessments. The timing of repeated instrumental assessment should be patient-specific and based on changes in symptoms rather than on an arbitrary amount of time between studies.[41–43]

SUMMARY

Neurologic dysphagia is enormously impactful not only for the medical health of the child affected but also for their social development, their quality of life, and the quality of life of their caregivers and loved ones. The treatment and management of neurologic dysphagia takes place over the long term, and this must be set as a clear expectation. Many children with neurologic dysphagia have multiple comorbidities, so it is crucial for care providers to practice joint decision-making with families. While some families may choose to follow the "safest" recommendations, others may choose to take the risk of PO intake in order to preserve the joy that eating and drinking can bring. Collaboration between medical specialties, therapists, and families can facilitate the best possible management of dysphagia for these complex patients.

CLINICS CARE POINTS

- Patients with neurologic dysphagia are frequently medically complex and may have multiple contributors to their swallowing dysfunction
- Use of instrumental swallowing studies in these populations can be helpful but should be ordered based on clinical changes rather than arbitrary ages or time intervals
- Management of patients with neurologic dysphagia should take a holistic approach and work toward each patient's unique goals of care

DISCLOSURE

The authors have no financial disclosures or conflicts of interest.

REFERENCES

1. Miller CK. Aspiration and swallowing dysfunction in pediatric patients. Infant Child Adolesc Nutr 2011;3(6):336–43.
2. Rudolph CD. Feeding disorders in infants and children. J Pediatr 1994;125(6): S116–24.
3. Dodrill P, Gosa MM. Pediatric dysphagia: physiology, assessment, and management. Ann Nutr Metabol 2015;66(Suppl. 5):24–31.
4. Ledford JR, Gast DL. Feeding problems in children with autism spectrum disorders: A review. Focus Autism Other Dev Disabil 2006;21(3):153–66.
5. Marshall J, Hill RJ, Ziviani J, et al. Features of feeding difficulty in children with Autism Spectrum Disorder. Int J Speech Lang Pathol 2014;16(2):151–8.
6. Slattery J, Morgan A, Douglas J. Early sucking and swallowing problems as predictors of neurodevelopmental outcome in children with neonatal brain injury: a systematic review. Dev Med Child Neurol 2012;54(9):796–806.
7. Kritzinger A, Krüger E, Pottas L. Breastfeeding and swallowing in a neonate with mild hypoxic-ischaemic encephalopathy. S Afr J Commun Disord 2017;64(1):1–7.
8. Krüger E, Kritzinger A, Pottas L. Oropharyngeal dysphagia in breastfeeding neonates with hypoxic-ischemic encephalopathy on therapeutic hypothermia. Breastfeed Med 2019;14(10):718–23.

9. Quattrocchi CC, Longo D, Delfino LN, et al. Dorsal brain stem syndrome: MR imaging location of brain stem tegmental lesions in neonates with oral motor dysfunction. Am J Neuroradiol 2010;31(8):1438–42.

10. Benfer KA, Weir KA, Bell KL, et al. Oropharyngeal dysphagia and gross motor skills in children with cerebral palsy. Pediatrics 2013;131(5):e1553–62.

11. Arvedson J. Feeding children with cerebral palsy and swallowing difficulties. Eur J Clin Nutr 2013;67(2):S9–12.

12. Rogers B, Arvedson J, Buck G, et al. Characteristics of dysphagia in children with cerebral palsy. Dysphagia 1994;9:69–73.

13. van den Engel-Hoek L, Erasmus CE, van Hulst KC, et al. Children with central and peripheral neurologic disorders have distinguishable patterns of dysphagia on videofluoroscopic swallow study. J Child Neurol 2014;29(5):646–53.

14. Adams RC, Elias ER, Disabilities COCW, et al. Nonoral feeding for children and youth with developmental or acquired disabilities. Pediatrics 2014;134(6): e1745–62.

15. Morgan A, Ward E, Murdoch B, et al. Incidence, characteristics, and predictive factors for dysphagia after pediatric traumatic brain injury. J Head Trauma Rehabil 2003;18(3):239–51.

16. Morgan AT. Dysphagia in childhood traumatic brain injury: a reflection on the evidence and its implications for practice. Dev Neurorehabil 2010;13(3):192–203.

17. Kilcommons A, Rawlinson D. Dysphagia and Long-Term Feeding Difficulties in the Pediatric Brain Tumor Population. Perspectives of the ASHA Special Interest Groups 2016;1(13):143–8.

18. Morgan AT, Sell D, Ryan M, et al. Pre and post-surgical dysphagia outcome associated with posterior fossa tumour in children. J Neurooncol 2008;87:347–54.

19. Audag N, Goubau C, Toussaint M, et al. Screening and evaluation tools of dysphagia in children with neuromuscular diseases: a systematic review. Dev Med Child Neurol 2017;59(6):591–6.

20. van den Engel-Hoek L, de Groot IJ, de Swart BJ, et al. Feeding and Swallowing Disorders in Pediatric Neuromuscular Diseases: An Overview. J Neuromuscul Dis 2015;2(4):357–69.

21. Van den Engel-Hoek L, Erasmus C, Van Bruggen H, et al. Dysphagia in spinal muscular atrophy type II: more than a bulbar problem? Neurology 2009;73(21): 1787–91.

22. Pane M, Vasta I, Messina S, et al. Feeding problems and weight gain in Duchenne muscular dystrophy. Eur J Paediatr Neurol 2006;10(5–6):231–6.

23. Elta GH, Caldwell CA, Nostrant TT. Esophageal dysphagia as the sole symptom in type I Chiari malformation. Dig Dis Sci 1996;41:512–5.

24. Hazkani I, Voyles C, Reddy KM, et al. The prevalence of Chiari malformation among children with persistent dysphagia. Am J Otolaryngol Jul-Aug 2023; 44(4):103887.

25. Petersson RS, Wetjen NM, Thompson DM. Neurologic variant laryngomalacia associated with Chiari malformation and cervicomedullary compression. Ann Otol Rhinol Laryngol 2011;120(2):99–103.

26. Pollack IF, Pang D, Kocoshis S, et al. Neurogenic dysphagia resulting from Chiari malformations. Neurosurgery 1992;30(5):709–19.

27. Albert GW, Menezes AH, Hansen DR, et al. Chiari malformation Type I in children younger than age 6 years: presentation and surgical outcome. J Neurosurg Pediatr 2010;5(6):554–61.

28. Putnam PE, Orenstein SR, Pang D, et al. Cricopharyngeal dysfunction associated with Chiari malformations. Pediatrics 1992;89(5):871–6.

29. Pomeraniec IJ, Ksendzovsky A, Awad AJ, et al. Natural and surgical history of Chiari malformation Type I in the pediatric population. J Neurosurg Pediatr 2016;17(3):343–52.

30. Faulks D, Collado V, Mazille MN, et al. Masticatory dysfunction in persons with Down's syndrome. Part 1: aetiology and incidence. J Oral Rehabil 2008;35(11): 854–62.

31. Jackson A, Maybee J, Moran MK, et al. Clinical characteristics of dysphagia in children with Down syndrome. Dysphagia 2016;31:663–71.

32. Stanley MA, Shepherd N, Duvall N, et al. Clinical identification of feeding and swallowing disorders in 0–6 month old infants with Down syndrome. Am J Med Genet 2019;179(2):177–82.

33. Jackson A, Maybee J, Wolter-Warmerdam K, et al. Associations between age, respiratory comorbidities, and dysphagia in infants with down syndrome. Pediatr Pulmonol 2019;54(11):1853–9.

34. Bull MJ, Trotter T, Santoro SL, et al. Genetics Co. Health supervision for children and adolescents with Down syndrome. Pediatrics 2022;149(5):e2022057010.

35. Erasmus CE, Van Hulst K, Van Den Hoogen FJ, et al. Thickened saliva after effective management of drooling with botulinum toxin A. Dev Med Child Neurol 2010; 52(6):e114–8.

36. Arvedson JC. Assessment of pediatric dysphagia and feeding disorders: clinical and instrumental approaches. Dev Disabil Res Rev 2008;14(2):118–27.

37. Freitag N, Tews P, Hübl N, et al. Laryngeal sensation and its association with aspiration and cough in children with neurological impairment. Pediatr Pulmonol 2021;56(12):3796–801.

38. Beer S, Hartlieb T, Müller A, et al. Aspiration in children and adolescents with neurogenic dysphagia: comparison of clinical judgment and fiberoptic endoscopic evaluation of swallowing. Neuropediatrics 2014;402–5.

39. Morton R, Minford J, Ellis R, et al. Aspiration with dysphagia: the interaction between oropharyngeal and respiratory impairments. Dysphagia 2002;17:192–6.

40. Arvedson J, Rogers B, Buck G, et al. Silent aspiration prominent in children with dysphagia. Int J Pediatr Otorhinolaryngol 1994;28(2–3):173–81.

41. Arvedson JCL-G, Maureen A. Pediatric videofluoroscopic swallow studies. A Professional Manual with Caregiver Guidelines. Communication Skill Builders/Psychological Corporation. San Antonio, TX; 1998. p. 106.

42. Arvedson JC, Lefton-Greif MA. Instrumental assessment of pediatric dysphagia. New York, NY: Thieme Medical Publishers; 2017. p. 135–46.

43. Martin-Harris B, Canon CL, Bonilha HS, et al. Best practices in modified barium swallow studies. Am J Speech Lang Pathol 2020;29(2S):1078–93.

Adult Esophageal Foreign Bodies

Mausumi Natalie Syamal, MD, MSE*

KEYWORDS

- Esophageal foreign body • Dysphagia • Esophageal food impaction

KEY POINTS

- Adult esophageal foreign bodies and food impactions present unique challenges and require special considerations in diagnosis, assessment, and management.
- Most impacted items require management as soon as possible or within 24 hours.
- Key to successful retrieval involves familiarity with a variety of endoscopes and retrieval instruments and often thinking "outside the box."

INTRODUCTION

Foreign body ingestion in adults poses unique challenges and requires special consideration. The otolaryngologist works in concert with gastroenterology, radoiology, anesthesiology, general/trauma, and thoracic surgery colleagues to treat these patients with urgency and efficiency. In a 2019 National Electronic Injury Surveillance System database survey, adult foreign body ingestions were found to have increased in incidence over the past 2 decades from 3 to 5.3 per 100,000 persons.[1] The survey revealed that age-specific incidence was bimodal with the adult peak in persons greater than 80 years of age with no specific difference in incidence between men and women.

Since the 1970s, it is believed that most esophageal foreign bodies will pass without incident leaving about 10% to 20% that will require nonoperative intervention, and less than 1% which require surgery.[2,3] While modern rates and mortality studies are absent in the literature, a 1976 study estimated that 1500 people die annually in the United States due to foreign body ingestion. Admissions for foreign body ingestion can be costly as they routinely require multispecialty consultations, imaging studies, endoscopic evaluation, observation, and the possibility of surgery with prolonged hospital admission. In a study comparing trends in adult esophageal foreign body hospital costs from 1998 to 2013, it was found that the rate of inpatient admissions has

Laryngology, Department of Otorhinolaryngology, Division of Laryngology, Rush University Medical Center, 1611 West Harrison Street, Suite 550, Chicago, IL 60612, USA
* Corresponding author.
E-mail address: Mausumi_N_Syamal@rush.edu

Otolaryngol Clin N Am 57 (2024) 609–621
https://doi.org/10.1016/j.otc.2024.01.003
0030-6665/24/© 2024 Elsevier Inc. All rights reserved.

decreased while the cost of these hospitalizations has increased with no change in surgical interventions for those patients.[4] For patients with deliberate foreign body ingestion, a 2010 review revealed the average cost was USD $11,000 per hospital admission.[5] Prompt recognition of the signs, symptoms, and the at-risk population during presentation is the key to ensuring quality-driven cost-effective treatment for these hospitalizations.

CLINICAL PRESENTATION & ETIOLOGY

Clinically the adult patient, if able to communicate well, will be able to report symptoms and recall the ingestion incident and the impacted substance. In a 2018 systematic review of impacted esophageal foreign bodies in adult patients, retrosternal pain (78%) followed by dysphagia (48%) and odynophagia (43.4%) were the most reported symptoms.[6] Respiratory symptoms were present in 4% and 3% of patients were asymptomatic.[6] Dysphonia or pharyngeal discomfort may also be present.[7] However, the area of discomfort does not always correlate to the site of impaction and is better the higher the object is impacted.[8] Additionally, if mental status is compromised, eliciting history from caregivers and loved ones about possible ingestion or impaction is the key. Asking about prior foreign body ingestions or food impactions is helpful. Patients with severe obstruction can present with hypersalivation, aspiration, and coughing, as well as the inability to tolerate secretions, neck swelling, erythema, tenderness, or crepitus (suggesting perforation).[9,10]

The clinical presentation may hinge upon whether the patient was aware of the possibility of ingestion and impaction. If the presenting symptom is vague, like globus, then asking about proximity of onset to meals or events is helpful. Esophageal food impaction is more likely to occur on American holidays and national athletic events and is associated with large meals.[11] Adults with either physiologic or anatomic narrowing of the esophagus are at higher risk of food or foreign body impaction after accidental or intentional ingestion of a foreign body and food bolus impaction.[12] Types of mechanical esophageal narrowing include esophageal strictures (most common), malignancy, esophageal webs or Schatzki's rings, or achalasia.[6,13] Functional narrowing includes adults with achalasia and esophageal spasm as well.[14] There have also been reports of increased incidence of food bolus obstruction in patients with eosinophilic esophagitis, likely due to pathologic changes such as mucosal rings and narrow bore esophagus.[15]

At-Risk/Vulnerable Populations

Adult esophageal foreign bodies can be separated into 3 categories: accidental/occult ingestion, deliberate ingestion, and food bolus impaction which may be either accidental or deliberate. Accidental ingestion is more common than deliberate.[16] Patients at high risk for deliberate impaction include body packers—people who drug smuggle in utilizing the gastrointestinal tract by swallowing different amounts of drugs, and those in police custody.[1]

Adults with mental or cognitive impairment and edentulous adults with dentures/dental protheses are also prone to foreign body ingestions.[1,9,17]

Deliberate, or intentional foreign body ingestion (DFBI) is the intentional ingestion of a true foreign body (a non-nutritional item) for self-injurious, parasuicidal reasons and accounts for approximately 14% of adult foreign body ingestions.[18] This often occurs in patients with underlying mental disorders such as Munchausen's by proxy, personality disorders, psychosis with delusions and hallucinations, malingering, pica,[19] and adults with intellectual impairments and neurodevelopment disorders such as *attention deficit hyperactivity disorder*, autism, and cerebral palsy. Malingering is often seen in adults who are institutionalized for long periods, such as inmates or those in mental health facilities. These behaviors are often resistant to intervention and are impulsive and repetitive.[20] Populations less studied, but nonetheless require consideration, are patients with binge eating disorders or patients who engage in competitive eating. **Box 1** summarizes the at-risk or vulnerable populations.

ASSESSMENT

Initial assessment involves assessing the severity of clinical symptoms and identifying the characteristics of the impacted foreign body. If airway security is in question, urgent/emergent measures should be taken to stabilize the airway. Patients unable to tolerate secretions with unstable vital signs require immediate airway management.[9] After a thorough clinical history and physical examination, imaging is generally obtained if the patient is stable. Biplane (antero-posterior and lateral view) radiographs identify most radiopaque materials and can identify free air, confirm the location, size, shape, and number of ingested foreign bodies as well as help exclude aspirated objects.[9] Radiographs are limited in their ability to identify fish or chicken bones, wood, plastic, glass, and thin metal objects thus, if these items are suspected, a computed tomography (CT) scan may be more useful.[9] Additionally, false positives may also occur due to the laryngeal calcifications along the styloid process or calcification of the stylohyoid ligament.[21] In a systematic review of esophageal perforations caused by edible foreign bodies, the diagnostic sensitivity of lateral neck X-rays was 56%, and CT scan was 100%.[3]

Swallowing studies should only be employed with extreme caution. If esophageal perforation is suspected, Gastrografin (meglucamine diatrizoate) swallow study is the most useful diagnostic swallow test since barium leakage risks mediastinitis.[22] However, Gastrografin is contraindicated in an obstructed esophagus because it is hypertonic and, if aspirated, it will cause pulmonary edema and severe pneumonitis.[14,23]

Box 1
Vulnerable adult populations

Elderly
    Edentulous with dental prostheses/dentures
    Dementia

Psychiatric disorders
    Munchausen's by proxy
    Personality disorders
    Psychosis with delusions and/or hallucinations
    Malingering
    Pica

Institutionalized adults

Intellectual or neurocognitively impaired adults

Binge eaters

Competitive eaters

Substance-associated
    Alcohol use/abuse
    Narcotic use
    Neurologically sedating medications
    Drug-packers

Both the American Society for Gastrointestinal Endoscopy and European Society of Gastrointestinal Endoscopy recommend against contrast swallows due to the risk of aspiration and worsening of the endoscopic visualization from coating.[9,10]

maging studies provide valuable information on the location of the foreign body which can determine whether other interventionalists should be involved. The cervical esophagus is the most common location for an impacted ingested foreign body.[6,24] Objects located proximal to the upper esophageal sphincter should be removed by an otolaryngologist as a laryngoscope is best suited for these retrievals.[14,23] An example being fishbones which are most commonly found in the oropharynx.[7]

TIMING OF INTERVENTION

As a rule of thumb, as Ginsberg aptly stated, "under no circumstances should a foreign object or food bolus impaction be allowed to remain in the esophagus beyond 24 hours from presentation."[14] Therefore, once radiological assessment has been completed, prompt identification and categorization of the suspected ingested material is paramount. This includes discerning between whether the object is edible or inedible and sharp versus blunt or an item of special concern (**Fig. 1**).

If the object is sharp like a bone (**Fig. 2**) or a nail, or glass, it should be removed as soon as possible (within 2 hours). Other emergent/urgent items include a disk or button battery, a magnet, any object larger than 2.5 cm in diameter, any object longer

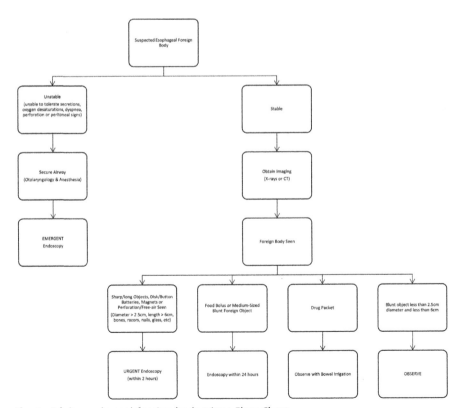

Fig. 1. Adult esophageal foreign body triage Flow Chart.

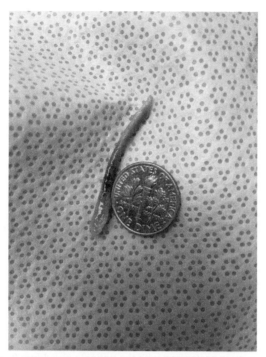

Fig. 2. Example of an adult ingested foreign body (bone) requiring urgent (within 2 hours) removal.

than 5 to 6 cm (difficulty passing the duodenum), or if the object is fully obstructing the esophagus, it is recommended that endoscopic retrieval be performed emergently, preferably within 2 hours.[9,10] Most common esophageal foreign bodies tend to be sharp which pose the highest risk of perforation (35%).[25] In a review of over 10,000 patients, the most common were sharp-pointed objects (38.1%) the majority of which were fish or chicken bones (80.7%)[6] The object impacted may be dependent on the region of the world or country as cuisines and dietary habits vary.

If the ingested body is small and blunt, and neither a disk battery nor a magnet, observation for passage is generally acceptable. There is literature supporting that intravenous glucagon (1 mg) may induce relaxation of the distal esophagus.[9,26,27] Other agents reported in the literature for possible assistance in passage include buscopan, oral nifedipine, and nitroglycerin,[6,28–30] Carbonated beverages have also been mentioned; however, in a multicentered randomized control trial, it did not have a meaningful effect on the improvement of food bolus obstruction.[31] Papain (Adolph's Meat Tenderizer) should not be given as it causes enzymatic degradation of the esophageal mucosal lining increasing risk of perforation and death[23,32]

If the ingested item is a drug packet, endoscopy and removal should be avoided as rupture of these packets often contain a lethal dose.[10,14,23] The European Society of Gastrointestinal Endoscopy strongly recommends that these patients undergo close clinical observation with bowel cleansing/irrigation, and radiographic follow-up for observing passage of the parcels. If a drug-packer patient is symptomatic, surgical intervention is recommended over endoscopy.[10] Serum and urine drug screens should be obtained to assess leakage and the patient should be admitted for inpatient observation.[14] **Fig. 1** summarizes general timing and management as described earlier.

MANAGEMENT

Management of an esophageal impacted or foreign body is through endoscopy. Gastroenterology literature more commonly employs flexible endoscopy, while otolaryngology literature advocates the use of rigid esophagoscopy as it is better for obstructions at or near the cricopharyngeus or for sharp objects.[24,30] In a 2018 meta-analysis of 736 flexible and 666 rigid esophagoscopy procedure for foreign body impaction, flexible and rigid were found to be equally safe for removal.[33] The method of extraction should take into consideration that flexible esophagoscopy is usually performed with local anesthesia with sedation while rigid requires general anesthesia with a secured airway. Additionally, the 2 methods may be complementary with rigid esophagoscopy often employed after flexible esophagoscopy failure or in challenging cases.[30]

Regardless of the scope employed, a variety of retrieval devices should be readily available when attempting extraction. Cupped, rat-toothed, and alligator forceps should be available. Thinking "outside the box" of one's specialty is helpful here as laparoscopic instruments (right angled instruments), overtubes, protector hoods, urologic balloons, biliary snares, and pediatric optical forceps can all be utilized.[34] If the object is identifiable, practice outside the patient with these instruments and a similar object (or replica) prior to beginning the procedure.[9]

Rigid esophagoscopy is performed with the patients shoulders flat on the table and head tilted upwards, the scope is held distally with the right hand and grasped proximally with the left and introduced "into the right pyriform sinus...lifting the larynx forward with the thumb of the left hand and directing the tip of the scope toward the suprasternal notch."[35] The cricopharyngeus will slowly relax and the scope can be inched forward slowly until the impacted object is seen. Depending on the grasping instrument, the esophagoscope may need to be regressed to allow for grasping room. Once grasp is secured, the esophagoscope should be advanced to contact the foreign body and forceps. All 3—foreign body, forceps, and esophagoscope— are gently withdrawn together.[35]

COMPLICATIONS

While most removal of esophageal foreign bodies proceed successfully, a surgical approach may be needed in about 3.4% because of unsuccessful endoscopic treatment, perforation, or fistula.[6] Aiolfi and colleagues found that 17.8% had a complication, with 1.4% perforation due to the foreign body and 0.3% iatrogenic perforation rate.[6,16] The mortality rate for perforations caused by edible foreign bodies is reported around 10%.[3] If a complication or perforation is suspected, CT imaging is an effective modality for diagnosing and managing the patient depending on the clinical picture.[3] Antibiotic therapy should be initiated promptly.[35] However, surgery may be inevitable when the patient is deteriorating, if foreign body was not found on endoscopy and/or perforation becomes evident, or if an aortoesophageal fistula is present.[24]

A study of 294 patients with esophageal foreign bodies found diabetes and duration of foreign body retention (>24 hr) independently increased risk for perforation.[36] Monitoring patients closely for fever, tachycardia, leukocytosis, and signs of sepsis under admission with strict nothing per oral administration is recommended if there are

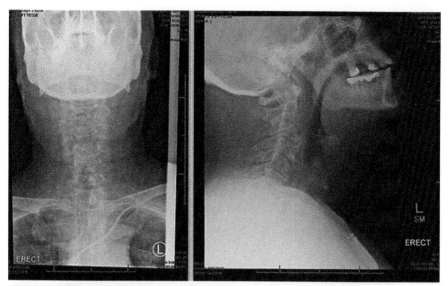

Fig. 3. Lateral and anteroposterior X-ray films did not reveal foreign body.

concerns for perforation or if extrication was difficult. The Pittsburgh perforation severity score links increasing clinical severity with several patient factors: age greater than 75, tachycardia, leukocytosis (>10, 000 WBC/mL), fever (>38.5°C), respiratory compromise (>30 respirations/min, increasing oxygen supplementation, or

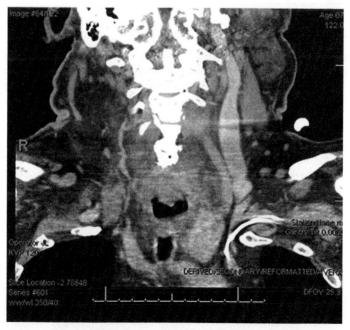

Fig. 4. Coronal computed tomography (CT) scan view revealing impacted esophageal foreign body.

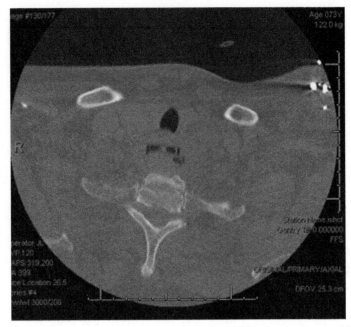

Fig. 5. Axial CT scan image revealing impacted esophageal foreign body resembling bottle cap described by the patient.

mechanical ventilation), leak seen on swallow/CT imaging, and the presence of cancer or hypotension are all score components.[37]

DISCUSSION

No discussion on esophageal foreign bodies can go without mention to Chevalier Jackson, who in his 1937 book meticulously documented 3266 cases of upper airway and esophageal foreign bodies, with 2600 photographs.[38] The observations and techniques outlined by Jackson are still utilized and relevant today. Presentation of an adult with an esophageal foreign body can be nuanced and the otolaryngologist is served well by acting promptly to piece together clinical clues with diagnostic information. Flexible laryngoscopy can be used to both determine the stability of the airway and to look for foreign bodies above the cricopharyngeus. When in doubt, a CT scan may reveal what is not easily seen on plain films. The following case illustrates

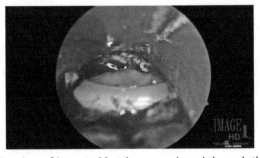

Fig. 6. Intraoperative view of impacted bottle cap as viewed through the esophagoscope.

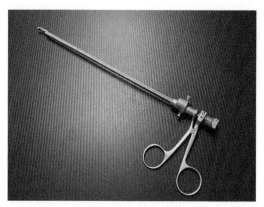

Fig. 7. Pediatric angled optical forceps (Olympus, Center Valley, PA).

the complex nature in which patients with esophageal foreign body present and illustrates several of the salient points within this section on management of the adult esophageal foreign body.

Case Presentation

A 73-year-old man was opening a plastic bottle of water with his mouth. The patient struggled with grip strength and so he was using his mouth. Relatives also reported that he was also prone to some memory issues. The bottle exploded upon opening and the resulting surprise caused him to reflexively swallow the cap of the bottle. He estimated that the cap measured approximately 0.5 cm × 1.5 cm. He had a brief choking/coughing episode after the initial event but improved quickly. He then tried performing self-Heimlich by throwing himself over the side of his couch. The patient also tried drinking soapy-water and grabbing the object with forceps but was unable to locate it. He then arrived at the emergency department where X-rays were taken (**Fig. 3**) which did not reveal a foreign body. Bedside flexible nasopharyngolaryngoscopy was negative and the patient was then discharged home.

Two days later, the patient returned to the emergency department now reporting worsening shortness of breath, chest discomfort, inability to tolerate liquids, and "gurgling" respirations. A CT was then performed (**Figs. 4** and **5**) which revealed an esophageal foreign body similar in appearance to the plastic bottle cap described by the patient.

The patient was then taken by the gastroenterology service for flexible endoscopy, necrotic tissue was noted and after 3 hours of attempted removal, the procedure was aborted. Next, the otolaryngologist was called in. As it was nearly midnight, calls were made pre-emptively to the Thoracic General Surgical services in the event an open surgical approach would be needed. An operating room was

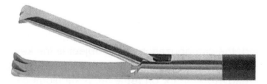

Fig. 8. 5-mm laparoscopic claw (Mediflex, Islandia, NY).

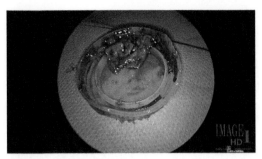

Fig. 9. Bottle cap once removed with necrotic mucosal tissue.

prepared with a variety of laryngeal and esophageal scopes and grasping instruments with a similar plastic bottle cap to practice. The patient was then brought into the operating room and intubated by anesthesia. A rigid oval esophagoscope 10 mm × 14 mm × 29 mm, length 291 mm was inserted (Piling, Fort Washington, PA) by the otolaryngologist, and slowly advanced keeping the lumen in view until the cap was identified (**Fig. 6**).

Pediatric angled optical forceps (Olympus, Center Valley, PA) were used as a right-angled pulling instrument (**Fig. 7**). The tip was advanced under the lip of the cap; the cap was then nudged forward while pulling scope backward until cap rested just below the cricopharyngeus. At the cricopharyngeus, the optical forceps were unable to securely grasp the cap to pull it out, so a 5-mm laparoscopic claw (Mediflex, Islandia, NY) was used to firmly grasp the cap and pull it out with the esophagoscope as a unit (**Fig. 8**).

Upon removal of the bottlecap, necrotic tissue was indeed noted on the cap (**Fig. 9**). A nasogastric tube was then placed under direct view through the rigid esophagoscope, and the patient was turned over to the general surgical team for placement of a gastric feeding tube. The patient was admitted and observed closely for signs of mediastinitis for several days. He was fed through his gastric tube. Repeat imaging and swallow greater than 72-h post-op confirmed no active-leak, and the patient eventually had his G-tube removed, resumed oral intake, and returned home.

SUMMARY

Foreign body ingestion or food bolus impaction is encountered frequently over the course of the career of an otolaryngologist in any setting. Special attention should be paid to the patient's mental status, noting possible substance abuse or intoxication. Prior history of foreign body impaction is also beneficial since the behavior may be recurrent in elderly, those with structural concerns (cancer or strictures) or those with secondary gain such as prisoners. While the nature of the impaction and item may vary based on geographic location or the population, the assessment and management remain nearly steadfast since the days of Chevalier Jackson. Prompt imaging with X-rays which are readily accessible provide a good first-line assessment whereas CT scans provide superior sensitivity to a wider range of objects. Once identified, the categorization of the object is the key to timely management as high-risk objects require intervention emergently or urgently. Once the otolaryngologist is ready to embark on retrieval, meticulous care should be taken to prepare and obtain all possible instruments for viewing and retrieving the object

safely which includes enlisting the help of surgical colleagues should be open techniques be required. During intervention, care should be taken to assess and prevent
perforation with a low threshold for observation and serial imaging if one is
suspected.

CLINICS CARE POINTS

- Adult esophageal foreign bodies have increased in incidence and may present with symptoms ranging from retrosternal pain and dysphagia to vague discomfort and globus.
- Adults with neurocognitive deficits, substance use history, or those who are incarcerated are considered some of the vulnerable populations prone to esophageal foreign bodies.
- CT scans have the highest sensitivity for diagnosis of foreign bodies.
- The most common adult esophageal foreign bodies are sharp bones located in the cervical esophagus.
- A prompt multidisciplinary approach is needed to identify and manage high-risk foreign bodies (sharp objects, button/disk batteries, magnets, objects larger than 2.5 cm or longer than 5–6 cm) or complete food impactions which require removal within 2 hours.
- Definitive management of less urgent foreign bodies or incomplete food impactions should be within 24 hours.
- Drug packets should not be retrieved endoscopically.
- The otolaryngologist should be skillful with the esophagoscope and with a wide variety of retrieval instruments across interventional specialties. Practicing with a replica of the object is strongly recommended prior to beginning intervention.
- There should be a low threshold for post-procedure admission and monitoring of complications (perforation) in cases where the foreign body was retained greater than 24 hours and in patients with diabetes, fever, tachycardia, hypotension, and leukocytosis.

REFERENCES

1. Hsieh A, Hsiehchen D, Layne S, et al. Trends and clinical features of intentional and accidental adult foreign body ingestions in the United States, 2000 to 2017. Gastrointest Endosc 2020;91(2):350–7.e1.
2. Schwartz GF, Polsky HS. Ingested foreign bodies of the gastrointestinal tract. Am Surg 1976;42(4):236–8.
3. Aronberg RM, Punekar SR, Adam SI, et al. Esophageal perforation caused by edible foreign bodies: A systematic review of the literature. Laryngoscope 2015;125:371–8.
4. Parikh MP, Garg R, Gupta N, et al. National trends in healthcare outcomes and utilization of endoscopic and surgical interventions in patients hospitalized with esophageal foreign body and food impaction. Dis Esophagus 2020. https://doi.org/10.1093/dote/doaa018. doaa018.
5. Huang BL, Rich HG, Simundson SE, et al. Intentional swallowing of foreign bodies is a recurrent and costly problem that rarely causes endoscopy complications. Clin Gastroenterol Hepatol 2010;8(11):941–6. https://doi.org/10.1016/j.cgh.2010.07.013.
6. Aiolfi A, Ferrari D, Riva CG, et al. Esophageal foreign bodies in adults: systematic review of the literature. Scand J Gastroenterol 2018;53(10–11):1171–8.

7. Herranz-Gonzalez J, Martinez-Vidal J, Garcia-Sarandeses A, et al. Esophageal Foreign Bodies in Adults. Otolaryngology-Head Neck Surg (Tokyo) 1991;105: 649–54.

8. Connolly AA, Birchall M, Walsh-Waring GP, et al. Ingested foreign bodies: patient guided localization is a useful clinical tool. Clin Otolaryngol 1992;17:520–4.

9. ASGE Standards of Practice Committee, Ikenberry SO, Jue TL, Anderson MA, et al. Management of ingested foreign bodies and food impactions. Gastrointest Endosc 2011;73(6):1085–91.

10. Birk M, Bauerfeind P, Deprez PH, et al. Removal of foreign bodies in the upper gastrointestinal tract in adults: European Society of Gastrointestinal Endoscopy (ESGE) Clinical Guideline. Endoscopy 2016;48(5):489–96.

11. Shuja A, Winston DM, Rahman AU, et al. Esophageal food impaction during cultural holidays and national athletic events. Gastroenterol Rep (Oxf). 2017; 5(1):43–6.

12. Ambe P, Weber SA, Schauer M, et al. Swallowed foreign bodies in adults. Dtsch Arztebl Int 2012;109(50):869–75.

13. Sung SH, Jeon SW, Son HS, et al. Factors predictive of risk for complications in patients with oesophageal foreign bodies. Dig Liver Dis 2011;43(8):632–5.

14. Ginsberg GG. Management of ingested foreign objects and food bolus impactions. Gastrointest Endosc 1995;41(1):33–8.

15. Kerlin P, Jones D, Remedios M, et al. Prevalence of eosinophilic esophagitis in adults with food bolus obstruction of the esophagus. J Clin Gastroenterol 2007; 41(4):356–61.

16. Wang X, Zhao J, Jiao Y, et al. Upper gastrointestinal foreign bodies in adults: A systematic review. Am J Emerg Med 2021;50:136–41.

17. Abdullah BJJ, Teong LK, Mahadevan J, et al. Dental prosthesis ingested and impacted in the esophagus and orolaryngopharynx. J Otolaryngol 1998;27: 190–4.

18. Kaazan P, Seow W, Tan Z, et al. Deliberate foreign body ingestion in patients with underlying mental illness: A retrospective multicentre study. Australas Psychiatry 2023;31(5):619–24.

19. Kamal I, Thompson J, Paquette DM. The hazards of vinyl glove ingestion in the mentally retarded patient with pica: new implications for surgical management. Can J Surg 1999;42(3):201–4.

20. Palta R, Sahota A, Bemarki A, et al. Foreign-body ingestion: characteristics and outcomes in a lower socioeconomic population with predominantly intentional ingestion. Gastrointest Endosc 2009;69(3 Pt 1):426–33.

21. Pinto A, Lanza C, Pinto F, et al. Role of plain radiography in the assessment of ingested foreign bodies in the pediatric patients. Semin Ultrasound CT MR 2015;36(1):21–7.

22. Michel L, Grillo HC, Malt RA. Esophageal perforation. Ann Thorac Surg 1982; 33(2):203–10.

23. Telford JJ. Management of ingested foreign bodies. Can J Gastroenterol 2005; 19(10):599–601.

24. Athanassiadi K, Gerazounis M, Metaxas E, et al. Management of esophageal foreign bodies: a retrospective review of 400 cases. Eur J Cardio Thorac Surg 2002;21(4):653–6.

25. Vizcarrondo FJ, Brady PG, Nord HJ. Foreign bodies of the upper gastrointestinal tract. Gastrointest Endosc 1983;29:208–10.

26. Ferruci TJ, Long JA. Radiologic treatment of esophageal food impaction using intravenous glucagon. Radiology 1977;125:25–8.

27. Trenkner SW, Maglinte D, Lehman GA, et al. Esophageal food impaction: treatment with glucagon. Radiology 1983;149:401.
28. Bell AF, Eibling DE. Nifedipine in the Treatment of Distal Esophageal Food Impaction. Arch Otolaryngol Head Neck Surg 1988;114(6):682–3.
29. Schimmel J, Slauson S. Swallowed Nitroglycerin to Treat Esophageal Food Impaction. Ann Emerg Med 2019;74(3):462–3.
30. Stubington TJ, Kamani T. Food bolus and oesophageal foreign body: a summary of the evidence and proposed management process. Eur Arch Oto-Rhino-Laryngol 2021;278(10):3613–23.
31. Tiebie EG, Baerends EP, Boeije T, et al. Efficacy of cola ingestion for oesophageal food bolus impaction: open label, multicentre, randomised controlled trial. BMJ 2023;383:e077294.
32. Holsinger JW, Furson RL, Sealy WC. Esophageal perforation following meat impaction and papain ingestion. JAMA 1968;204:188–9.
33. Ferrari D, Aiolfi A, Bonitta G, et al. Flexible versus rigid endoscopy in the management of esophageal foreign body impaction: systematic review and meta-analysis. World J Emerg Surg 2018;13:42.
34. Nelson DB, Bosco JJ, Curtis W, et al. Endoscopic retrieval devices. Gastrointest Endosc 1999;50:932–4.
35. Jackson CL. Foreign bodies in the esophagus. Am J Surg 1957;93(2):308–12.
36. Zhang S, Wen J, Du M, et al. Diabetes is an independent risk factor for delayed perforation after foreign bodies impacted in esophagus in adults. United European Gastroenterol J 2018;6(8):1136–43.
37. Schweigert M, Sousa HS, Solymosi N, et al. Spotlight on esophageal perforation: A multinational study using the Pittsburgh esophageal perforation severity scoring system. J Thorac Cardiovasc Surg 2016;151(4):1002–9.
38. Diseases of the air and food passages of foreign body Origin. By Chevalier J., Sc.D. and CL. Jackson, A.B., M.D. W. B. Saunders & Co., Ltd., Philadelphia and London. 1936, 969 52s. 6d.

Pediatric Esophageal Foreign Bodies and Caustic Ingestions

Kristina Powers, MD[a], Cristina Baldassari, MD[b],
Jordyn Lucas, MD[b],*

KEYWORDS

- Esophageal foreign body ingestions • Caustics ingestions • Diagnostic testing
- Operative techniques • Pediatrics

KEY POINTS

- Foreign body ingestions are most common in children aged under 6 years. Sharp objects, button batteries, caustic substances, and multiple magnets should raise concern for more severe complications.
- Factors such as type and location of object, time since ingestion, and patient symptoms should be considered to guide treatment.
- Caustic ingestions, which are typically of household substances, can lead to long-term complications such as stricture.

INTRODUCTION: FOREIGN BODY INGESTIONS

Foreign body ingestions are an increasingly prevalent problem in the pediatric population.[1] Children with psychiatric diagnoses, developmental delay, and those aged under 6 years are most frequently affected.[1,2] Objects found around the home are most commonly ingested. Propensity to place things in their mouths, underdeveloped swallow reflexes, and incomplete molars contribute to ingestion.[1,3] Coins are the most common objects followed by toys, jewelry, and batteries in the United States.[2] Symptoms range from completely asymptomatic to respiratory distress, dysphagia, chest pain, and drooling.[4] Although most foreign bodies pass through the gastrointestinal (GI) tract without complications, problems can arise depending on the type of object ingested.[5,6] Overall, aerodigestive foreign bodies make up 1000 pediatric deaths per year.[3]

Unwitnessed events comprise a majority of foreign body ingestions. Annually over 100,000 emergency room visits are due to foreign body ingestions.[7] A recent study

[a] Department of Otolaryngology–Head and Neck Surgery, Eastern Virginia Medical School, Norfolk, VA, USA; [b] Department of Otolaryngology–Head and Neck Surgery, Eastern Virginia Medical School, Children's Hospital of the King's Daughters, Norfolk, VA, USA
* Corresponding author. 600 Gresham Drive #1100, Norfolk, VA 23507.
E-mail address: Jordyn.Lucas@chkd.org

Otolaryngol Clin N Am 57 (2024) 623–633
https://doi.org/10.1016/j.otc.2024.02.016
0030-6665/24/© 2024 Elsevier Inc. All rights reserved.

showed that the annual foreign body ingestion rate increased 91.5% in a 20 year period from 1995 to 2015.[2] Numerous studies have illustrated the effect of the coronavirus disease 2019 pandemic on foreign body ingestion and showed an increase in the incidence of dangerous ingestions such as button batteries and magnets, likely because children were home more often.[8,9] Additionally, there was a significant increase in ingestions in older children during this time.[9]

Only 10% of children presenting to the emergency room with foreign body ingestions are admitted to the hospital but over 80% of these children undergo a treatment intervention such as endoscopy.[2,10] The idea of foreign body removal dates back to the early 1900s when Chevalier Jackson began using instrumentation with improved visualization to remove foreign bodies. He was credited with the title, "the father of endoscopic aerodigestive foreign body removal" in addition to passing an act to require labeling of caustic chemicals to reduce ingestion in 1927. Since then, other laws have been passed which require labeling and secure packaging on many high-risk products. Parental counseling regarding age-appropriate toys and food pieces is vital in reducing adverse outcomes from ingestion.[3]

BUTTON BATTERIES

Button battery ingestions can result in serious harm to children. Lithium batteries are especially dangerous because they react with saliva to produce an electrical current leading to caustic injury as soon as 2 hours following ingestion. This can occur even when batteries are dead.[3] Button batteries larger than 20 mm are associated with poorer outcomes due to their propensity to lodge in the upper esophageal sphincter.[3,11] This can lead to severe tissue damage and delayed complications such as perforation and fistulization into major blood vessels or the trachea, which can potentially result in death.[12] As the 20 mm lithium button batteries are used more frequently in various household products including toys, the number of severe complications and fatalities increased 6.7 fold in the past 25 years. Prompt recognition and diagnosis is crucial in these children.[11,12] Due to this increasing incidence and its impact on public health, mitigation strategies are being developed including public awareness campaigns and legislative regulation.[7] A promising new strategy called quantum tunneling composite coating involves a button battery that is only functional when pressure greater that the human body is capable of producing is applied to the battery.[12] A collaborative button battery task force was created in 2012, which implemented repackaging with the addition of warning labels.[13] Despite these interventions, rates of ingestion and complications continue to increase and more public awareness and mitigation strategies are necessary.[12,13]

COINS

Coin ingestions account for up to 80% of all foreign body ingestions and are most common in children aged 1 to 3 years.[1,7] Younger children have higher hospitalization and complication rates.[14] Because coins are blunt and inert, they typically do not cause significant complications unless they become lodged and lead to obstruction.[7] Once the coin enters the stomach, it is likely to pass without intervention.[7] Coins can often be mistaken as button batteries so imaging to differentiate the two is vital to guide management.[1]

MAGNETS

Magnet ingestions are typically seen in a biphasic peak with toddlers commonly swallowing magnetic toys and teenagers accidently swallowing fake magnetic tongue and lip piercings.[15] Magnets are dangerous when multiple are ingested as they can attach to each other in the GI tract causing necrosis, perforation, and fistulization of the tissue.[1,16] When single magnets are ingested, it is important to avoid magnets in the surrounding environment such as clothing.[16] It is critical to differentiate between single and multiple magnet ingestion with imaging to guide management. A new magnet composed of neodymium, iron, and boron and is 10 to 20 times stronger than a standard magnet has been recalled in numerous countries. This magnet is highly dangerous and has the potential to cause perforation in up to 50% of ingestions within 12 to 48 hours.[15] Proper parental education and public health initiatives are necessary to reduce the incidence of magnet ingestions.

FOOD

Esophageal food impaction is more common in adults; however, comorbidities such as eosinophilic esophagitis, anatomic obstructions, and disorders of decreased motility increase the risk in children.[4] This is a diagnostic challenge because food is organic and therefore radiolucent on standard radiographs.[17] Point-of-care ultrasonography has been proposed as a method to visualize food impaction while reducing the risk of radiation.[17] Food impaction should raise suspicion for an underlying esophageal disorder and biopsies of the esophagus should be considered if endoscopic removal is pursued.[18]

OTHERS

Superabsorbent polymer toy ingestions, marketed as Orbeez (Orbeez.co© 2024), have been increasing in recent years and grow when ingested leading to obstruction.[19] Sharp objects including fragments of metal and glass, fish bones, needles, and pins have the potential to traumatize or perforate the mucosa.[1,6,20] Swallowing drug-filled packets also known as "body packing" has increased worldwide over the past 30 years. Mortality is often times due to accidental ingestion and overdose from a ruptured packet. Surgical removal is indicated in cases of obstruction, perforation, symptoms of drug toxicity, or prolonged retention due to fear of inducing a toxic rupture.[21]

DISCUSSION: FOREIGN BODY INGESTIONS
Typical Clinical Presentation

- The most common scenario is an asymptomatic child brought to medical attention following a witnessed ingestion.
- Thorough head and neck examination to rule out foreign bodies in other locations such as the ears or nose.[7]

If unwitnessed, presenting symptoms are often nonspecific, physical examination warning signs include

- Crepitus, swelling, or erythema of the neck or chest can be indicative of foreign body with perforation.
- Abdominal findings such as rebound tenderness, guarding, and rigidity indicate peritonitis secondary to perforation.[1]

Workup

Plain film radiograph

- Routinely the first diagnostic step and recommended even in the absence of symptoms if foreign body ingestion is suspected.[6,7]

- Anteroposterior (AP) and lateral films of the neck, chest, and abdomen are most commonly used.[7] The positive predictive value of radiographic identification of metallic objects is 100% and much lower for radiolucent objects such as fish bones, wood, and glass[4] (**Table 1**).
- Round, flat objects such as coins or button batteries are characteristically en face on AP films and linear on lateral imaging as seen in **Fig. 1**A, B.[7] This is opposite of round, flat objects in the airway which would be linear on AP imaging and en face on lateral imaging.[1]
- An important differentiation between coins and button batteries is the "double ring" or "halo" sign anteriorly or a "2 layer" or "step-off sign" laterally on a button battery image (**Fig. 1**C, D).[1,7]
- Tracheal compression, tracheal deviation, esophageal air trapping, or bowel obstruction may be present if the object is not visible.

Other imaging modalities

- *Computed tomography (CT)* is used to assess for radiolucent objects[1,7] (**Fig. 2**).
- *MRI* is typically not indicated in the initial workup but can be useful when following a patient for complications after foreign body removal, especially in button battery ingestion.[4]
- *Upper GI studies with contrast* have the potential to precisely locate radiolucent objects; however, there is a concern with this delaying treatment.[4] This test is also user dependent and can fail to evaluate and diagnose other causes of a patient's symptoms.[24]
- *Ultrasonography* has been shown to successfully localize both radiopaque and radiolucent upper esophageal foreign bodies (**Fig. 3**).[25,26]

Treatment

Factors taken into account when deciding on the removal of esophageal foreign bodies include time since ingestion, symptoms, location in the esophagus, patient's age, and object ingested. Lower risk items, such as coins, can be given a trial of observation.[27–29] About 25% to 30% of asymptomatic children with esophageal coin ingestion were shown to have spontaneous passage within 24 hours.[28] Upon passage of a coin into the stomach of a healthy child, it will almost always pass through the remainder of the GI tract without further issue.[29] Spontaneous passage of coins was more common in older patients and more likely to occur when the coin was in the distal one-third of the esophagus (56% vs 27%).[28] Symptoms are more likely to be associated with the presence of a coin that does not pass within 24 hours.[30] These findings and observational studies suggest an observation period of somewhere between 8 and 16 hours with repeat radiograph prior to proceeding with endoscopic removal especially among older asymptomatic children with distally located coins.[27,31] Higher risk items such as sharp

Table 1	
Radiopaque and radiolucent objects[1,19,22,23]	
Radiopaque	**Radiolucent**
Coins	Wood
Metals	Plastic
Button batteries	Glass
Magnets	Fish bones
Medications: Iron, potassium chloride, amiodarone, spironolactone,	Food
bisoprolol, and lisinopril	Polymers

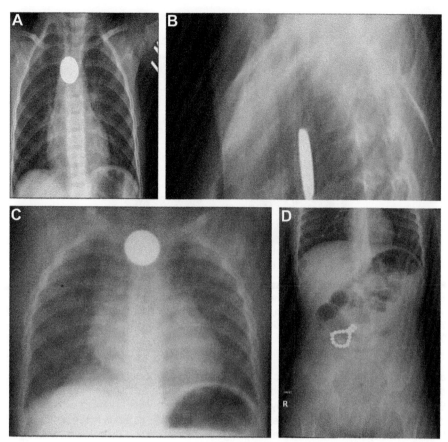

Fig. 1. Radiographs of common foreign bodies ingested by children. (*A*) AP view of button battery in the esophagus. (*B*) Lateral view of button battery in the esophagus. (*C*) AP view of coin in the esophagus. (*D*) AP view of multiple magnets in the small intestines. (Altokhais T (2021) Magnet Ingestion in Children Management Guidelines and Prevention. Front. Pediatr. 9:727988. https://doi.org/10.3389/fped.2021.727988)

objects, organic material due to the tendency to absorb fluid, material with oils that can cause further mucosal inflammation, and button batteries require a more urgent approach to removal.

Endoscopic removal

General anesthesia with endotracheal intubation occurs in 90% of cases of esophageal foreign body removal reported.[27] Endotracheal intubation prevents aspiration of gastric contents and provides a safe airway to allow sufficient time for removal.[32] Objects sitting in the cervical esophagus or postcricoid region of the larynx may be removed by direct laryngoscopy using the Magill forceps once the airway is secured with an endotracheal tube.

Esophagoscopy, rigid or flexible, is used to retrieve esophageal foreign bodies in the majority of cases.[33] Advantages of both rigid and flexible esophagoscopy include visualization of the object and the ability to further examine the mucosa and esophagus for damage.[31] Success rates of foreign body retrieval using rigid endoscopy have been reported at 95.4% and 97.4% with flexible esophagoscopy, with no significant

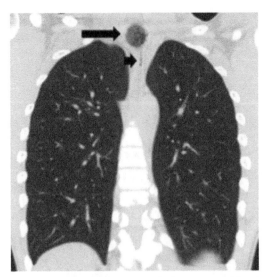

Fig. 2. Coronal noncontrast CT chest showing a radiolucent round foreign body, which was found to be a plastic bottle cap in the esophagus (*small arrow*) with trapped air above (*large arrow*). (*From* Marla, J. Herman Kan, Somcio R, et al. Chest CT for the Diagnosis of Pediatric Esophageal Foreign Bodies. 2021;50(5):566-570. https://doi.org/10.1067/j.cpradiol.2021.03. 012.)

difference in a recent systematic review. Commonly reported surgical risks include damage to lips or teeth and mucosal injury with esophageal perforation being rare.[34] Esophagoscope choice is usually specialty dependent. When dealing with sharp or penetrating foreign bodies, rigid endoscopy may be advantageous in removal by protecting the object and in turn the esophageal mucosa. When using rigid esophagoscopy, there are various instruments that can aid in retrieval, including a rat tooth grasper and peanut grasper. Other devices that can aid in retrieval when performing flexible esophagoscopy include a net retriever, overtubes, grasping device, rotatable retrieval basket, and foreign body snare.[35]

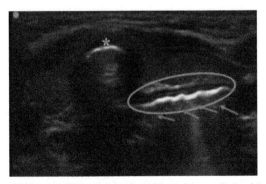

Fig. 3. Ultrasound of upper esophagus showing a linear hyperechoic object within the circle suggestive of a coin with artifact shown by the arrows. The *asterick* is the trachea. (*From* Mori T, Nomura O, Hagiwara Y. Another Useful Application of Point-of-Care Ultrasound. Pediatric Emergency Care. 2019; 35 (2): 154-156. https://doi.org/10.1097/PEC.0000000000001729.)

Bougienage and Foley catheter

Bougienage is a procedure in which a bougie dilator is passed through the oral cavity into the esophagus with the goal of passing the object into the stomach and allowing for the object to be passed naturally. This method is typically reserved for uncomplicated coin ingestions and used primarily by either pediatric surgeons or emergency room physicians. Success rates have been reported at 94%.[36] A Foley catheter can also be passed distal to a blunt foreign body and carefully removed with the foreign body after inflating the balloon. Success rates have been reported at greater than 85% with few adverse effects.[37] While these techniques may not require general anesthesia, there is a risk of aspiration.

Button battery management

Button battery ingestion is a medical emergency and requires emergent removal in the operating room. A recently developed button battery management protocol details the utility of honey (in children aged older than 1 year) or sucralfate that can be administered orally for ingestions that have occurred in less than 12 hours by caregivers, first responders, or emergency room personnel. However, administration of these substances should not delay emergent endoscopic surgical removal. Care should be taken to thoroughly examine the esophageal mucosa during removal and determine the location and direction of the negative pole of the battery to anticipate potential complications. If there is no esophageal perforation, the esophageal mucosa at the site the battery was lodged should be irrigated with acetic acid. Airway evaluation in the operating room, including direct laryngoscopy and bronchoscopy, should also be considered in cases with evidence of extensive esophageal mucosal injury. The full extent of injury may not be apparent in batteries that were more recently ingested. Thus, a repeat endoscopy at least 48 to 72 hours after injury may be considered. Complications include tracheoesophageal fistulas, esophageal strictures, mediastinitis, vocal cord paralysis, or spondylodiscitis.[38,39] The majority of complications present in a delayed manner (greater than 30 days following presentation with initial ingestion), so close follow-up of these patients is warranted.

Caustics

Caustic substances are typically composed of strong acids or bases that cause immediate harm to tissue after direct contact. They occur in a bimodal distribution consisting of accidental ingestion in children aged under 5 years and suicide attempts in adolescents and adults.[1] Commonly ingested agents include drain or other household cleaners (50%), bleach (30%–40%), and laundry detergent (20%). Approximately 3.7% of patients experience major complications and 0.02% deaths have been shown to be associated with household ingestions. The mechanism of injury is related to the concentration and pH of the ingested substance.[40] Ingestion of strong bases with pH greater than 11 can cause severe liquefactive necrosis leading to potential deep injury and perforation with possible thrombosis of surrounding vessels leading to reduced healing. Ingestion of bases with a lower pH rarely causes serious injuries. Ingestion of strong acids results in coagulation necrosis that can cause obstruction or perforation most commonly associated with gastric injury.[40,41] Long-term, untreated caustic ingestions can cause fibrosis leading to dysphagia.[41] Common presenting symptoms include vomiting, dysphagia, odynophagia, chest pain, dyspnea, abdominal pain, voice change, and tachycardia with vomiting.[1,41] Initial evaluation should focus on the type, volume, and timing of the ingestion if witnessed.[4] Consider flexible fiberoptic evaluation of the airway to assess for upper airway edema. The patient should be stabilized with potential intubation or surgical airway management if necessary.[41] A treatment algorithm for caustic ingestions is shown in **Fig. 4**. Intentional vomiting is not recommended as a treatment option as it reintroduces the caustic substance to the esophagus.[3]

The timing of endoscopy is favored between 12 and 24 hours following ingestion to reduce missing an early lesion or causing perforation later on. Many studies have shown an increase in complications such as stricture formation following steroid use. Antibiotics have no convincing evidence to support routine use unless patients are at risk for esophageal perforation.[3,40] Patients must be closely followed to evaluate

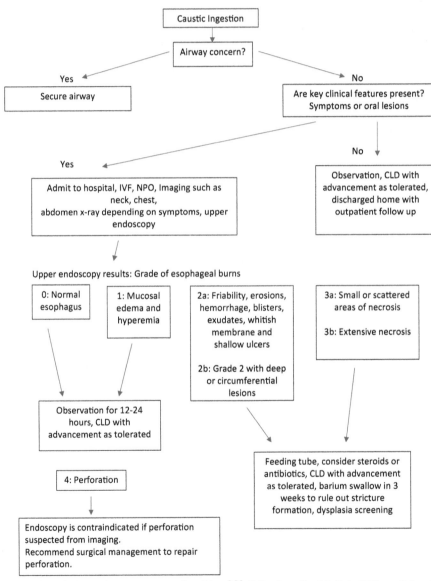

Fig. 4. Caustic ingestion treatment algorithm.[3,26] CLD, clear liquid diet; NPO, nothing by mouth.

for stricture formation as the risk of stricture is positively correlated with esophageal burn grade with nearly 100% of grade III patients developing stricture. Strictures are typically seen by 8 weeks in 80% of patients developing stricture.[40,41] Supraglottic stenosis can also occur, so close follow-up in patients with upper airway involvement is warranted. Another long-term complication is the development of esophageal carcinoma. If a severe caustic ingestion occurred, it is recommended to screen for dysplasia.[40]

SUMMARY

Overall, it is important to note whether ingested items are high risk for complications and poor outcomes. Chest radiographs are important in diagnosis, with advances being made with other imaging techniques such as ultrasonography. Timing, location, and presence of symptoms help to determine whether endoscopic removal with rigid or flexible esophagoscopy is needed. Ingested button batteries require emergent evaluation with immediate removal when lodged in the esophagus. Caustic ingestions can lead to strictures, and proper timing of esophagoscopy is important in the diagnosis and management of sequela.

CLINICS CARE POINTS

- Obtaining a thorough history and physical examination followed by plain film radiographs are the first steps in evaluation.
- If a foreign body ingestion was witnessed or suspected without evidence on radiographs, radiolucent objects should be considered and worked up with further imaging modalities.
- Treatment of foreign bodies consists of a wait-and-watch approach for coins in some patient populations and operative intervention for the removal of higher risk ingestions and coins that do not pass within 24 hours.
- Rigid esophagoscopy, flexible esophagoscopy, bougienage, and Foley catheter are all options for removal.
- Button battery ingestion is a medical emergency. Early operative removal is imperative for batteries lodged in the esophagus.
- For patients with symptoms or oral lesions after caustic ingestion, upper endoscopy within 12 to 24 hours should be performed to determine the grade of esophageal burn to guide further management.
- Barium swallow 3 weeks following severe injury after ingestion to evaluate for stricture and also monitor for dysplasia long term in patients with a history of severe caustic injuries.

DISCLOSURE

The authors have no relevant financial disclosures or conflicts of interest to report.

REFERENCES

1. Norris N, Barth B. *Foreign Body Ingestion in Children.* ed. Elsevier; 2023.
2. Orsagh-Yentis D, McAdams RJ, Roberts KJ, et al. Foreign-Body Ingestions of Young Children Treated in US Emergency Departments: 1995–2015. Pediatrics 2019;143(5):e20181988.
3. Schoem SR, Rosbe KW, Lee ER. Aerodigestive foreign bodies and caustic ingestions. *Cummings Pediatric Otolaryngology.* Elsevier; 2021. p. 483–96.

4. Kramer RE, Lerner DG, Lin T, et al. Management of Ingested Foreign Bodies in Children. J Pediatr Gastroenterol Nutr 2015;60(4):562–74.
5. Lee JH. Foreign Body Ingestion in Children. Clinical Endoscopy 2018;51(2): 129–36.
6. Conners GP and Mohseni M. Pediatric foreign body ingestion. PubMed, Available at: https://www.ncbi.nlm.nih.gov/books/NBK430915/, 2020. Accessed December 22, 2023.
7. Joyamaha D, Conners GP. Managing Pediatric Foreign Body Ingestions. Mo Med 2015;112(3):181–6.
8. Neal JT, Monuteaux MC, Porter JJ, et al. The Effect of COVID-19 Stay-At-Home Orders on the Rate of Pediatric Foreign Body Ingestions. J Emerg Med 2022; 63(6):729–37.
9. Geibel E, Pasman E, Nylund C, et al. The Impact of the COVID-19 Pandemic on Foreign Body Ingestion Trends in Children: A Comparison of the Pre-Pandemic Period to 2020. J Pediatr Gastroenterol Nutr 2022;75(3):299–303.
10. Wood ML, Potnuru PP, Nair S. Inpatient Pediatric Foreign Body Ingestion: National Estimates and Resource Utilization. J Pediatr Gastroenterol Nutr 2021; 73(1):37–41.
11. Varga Á, Kovács T, Saxena AK. Analysis of Complications After Button Battery Ingestion in Children. Pediatr Emerg Care 2018;34(6):443–6.
12. Litovitz T, Whitaker N, Clark L. Preventing battery ingestions: an analysis of 8648 cases. Pediatrics 2010;125(6):1178–83.
13. Eck JB, Ames WA. Anesthetic Implications of Button Battery Ingestion in Children. Anesthesiology 2020;1. https://doi.org/10.1097/aln.0000000000003121.
14. Chen X, Milkovich SM, Stool D, et al. Nicole Rider. Pediatric coin ingestion and aspiration. Int J Pediatr Otorhinolaryngol 2006;70(2):325–9.
15. Seguier-Lipszyc E, Samuk I, Almog A, et al. Multiple magnet ingestion in children: A problem on the rise. J Paediatr Child Health 2022;58(10):1824–8.
16. Hussain SZ, Bousvaros A, Gilger M, et al. Management of ingested magnets in children. J Pediatr Gastroenterol Nutr 2012;55(3):239–42.
17. Mori T, Ihara T, Hagiwara Y. Pediatric food impaction detected through point-of-care ultrasonography. Clinical and Experimental Emergency Medicine 2018; 5(2):135–7.
18. Hurtado CW, Furuta GT, Kramer RE. Etiology of Esophageal Food Impactions in Children. J Pediatr Gastroenterol Nutr 2011;52(1):43–6.
19. Caré W, Dufayet L, Paret N, et al. Bowel obstruction following ingestion of super-absorbent polymers beads: literature review. Clin Toxicol 2021;60(2):159–67.
20. Quitadamo Paolo, Battagliere Ilaria, Margherita Del Bene, et al. Sharp-Pointed Foreign Body Ingestion in Pediatric Age. J Pediatr Gastroenterol Nutr 2022; 76(2):213–7.
21. Kucukmetin NT, Gucyetmez B, Poyraz T, et al. Foreign material in the gastrointestinal tract: cocaine packets. Case Rep Gastroenterol 2014;8(1):56–60.
22. Uyemura MC. Foreign body ingestion in children. Am Fam Physician 2005;72(2): 287–91 [published correction appears in Am Fam Physician. 2006 Apr 15;73(8): 1332].
23. Dhruv S, Atodaria KP, Seog WJ, et al. Ingested Potassium Chloride Pills on Imaging Misdiagnosed As Foreign Bodies in the Stomach: An Insight on Radiopaque/Hyperdense Substances in the Gastrointestinal Tract. Cureus 2022. https://doi.org/10.7759/cureus.27116.
24. Marla J, Herman K, Somcio R, et al. Chest CT for the Diagnosis of Pediatric Esophageal Foreign Bodies 2021;50(5):566–70.

25. Mori T, Nomura O, Hagiwara Y. Another Useful Application of Point-of-Care Ultrasound. Pediatr Emerg Care 2019;35(2):154–6.
26. Hosokawa T, Yamada Y, Sato Y, et al. Role of Sonography for Evaluation of Gastrointestinal Foreign Bodies. J Ultrasound Med 2016;35(12):2723–32.
27. Crysdale WS, Sendi KS, Yoo J. Esophageal foreign bodies in children. 15-year review of 484 cases. Ann Otol Rhinol Laryngol 1991;100(4 Pt 1):320–4.
28. Waltzman ML, Baskin M, Wypij D, et al. A randomized clinical trial of the management of esophageal coins in children. Pediatrics 2005;116(3):614–9.
29. Schunk JE, Corneli H, Bolte R. Pediatric coin ingestions. A prospective study of coin location and Symptoms. Am J Dis Child 1989;5.
30. Caravati EM, Bennett DL, Mcelwee NE. Pediatric Coin Ingestion: A Prospective Study on the Utility of Routine Roentgenograms. Am J Dis Child 1989;143(5):549–51.
31. Conners GP, Chamberlain JM, Ochsenschlager DW. Conservative management of pediatric distal esophageal coins. J Emerg Med 1996;14(6):723–6.
32. Rodríguez H, Passali GC, Gregori D, et al. Management of foreign bodies in the airway and oesophagus. Int J Pediatr Otorhinolaryngol 2012;76(SUPPL. 1).
33. Yalçin Ş, Karnak I, Ciftci AO, et al. Foreign body ingestion in children: an analysis of pediatric surgical practice. Pediatr Surg Int 2007;23(8):755–61.
34. Yang W, Milad D, Wolter NE, et al. Systematic review of rigid and flexible esophagoscopy for pediatric esophageal foreign bodies. Int J Pediatr Otorhinolaryngol 2020;139.
35. Rammohan R, Joy M, Natt D, et al. Navigating the Esophagus: Effective Strategies for Foreign Body Removal. Cureus 2023;15(5).
36. Heinzerling NP, Christensen MA, Swedler R, et al. Safe and effective management of esophageal coins in children with bougienage. Surgery 2015;158(4):1065–72.
37. Choe JY, Choe BH. Foreign Body Removal in Children Using Foley Catheter or Magnet Tube from Gastrointestinal Tract. Pediatr Gastroenterol Hepatol Nutr 2019;22(2):132–41.
38. Jatana KR, Litovitz T, Reilly JS, et al. Pediatric button battery injuries: 2013 task force update. Int J Pediatr Otorhinolaryngol 2013;77(9):1392–9.
39. Mubarak A, Benninga MA, Broekaert I, et al. Diagnosis, Management, and Prevention of Button Battery Ingestion in Childhood: A European Society for Paediatric Gastroenterology Hepatology and Nutrition Position Paper. J Pediatr Gastroenterol Nutr 2021;73(1):129–36.
40. Kay M, Wyllie R. Caustic ingestions in children. Curr Opin Pediatr 2009;21(5):651–4.
41. Baskin D, Urganci N, Abbasoğlu L, et al. A standardised protocol for the acute management of corrosive ingestion in children. Pediatr Surg Int 2004;20(11–12):824–8.

Dysphagia in Head and Neck Cancer

Deepak Lakshmipathy, BS[a], Melissa Allibone, MS, CCC-SLP[a,b],
Karthik Rajasekaran, MD[a,c],*

KEYWORDS

- Dysphagia • Head and neck cancer • Swallowing • Nutrition

KEY POINTS

- Evaluation for dysphagia in patients with head and neck cancer must consider both the neoplasm and associated treatments as contributory factors.
- Patient-centered goals of care should dictate management.
- Prevention of dysphagia is an invaluable form of care alongside supportive treatments, swallowing therapies, and interventional measures.
- A variety of subjective and objective metrics exist to assess clinical outcomes of dysphagia and can guide management.

INTRODUCTION/HISTORY/DEFINITIONS/BACKGROUND

Head and neck (HN) cancers broadly refer to cancers of the upper aerodigestive tract.[1] Intuitively, their anatomic location can often lead to dysphagia in afflicted patients from both disease progression and involved treatments. The heterogeneity of tumor subtypes and affected populations makes approximating epidemiology of associated dysphagia difficult; however, some recent estimates report up to 100% prevalence among sampled patients.[2] The most common type of dysphagia affecting patients with HN cancer is pharyngeal dysphagia.[2,3] Specifically, these patients often have difficulty with the onset of swallowing, leading to possible aspiration and inability to transfer boluses along the oropharyngeal and gastrointestinal tracts. Timely evaluation and appropriate treatment are therefore critical to prevent unwanted sequelae.[2,3]

Management of dysphagia in patients with HN cancer involves a complex balance between ensuring good quality of life (QOL), respecting patient wishes, and

[a] Department of Otorhinolaryngology–Head & Neck Surgery, University of Pennsylvania, 800 Walnut Street, 18th Floor, Philadelphia, PA 19107, USA; [b] Department of Speech-Language Pathology, University of Pennsylvania, 800 Walnut Street, 18th Floor, Philadelphia, PA 19107, USA; [c] Leonard Davis Institute of Health Economics, University of Pennsylvania, 3641 Locust Walk, Philadelphia, PA 19104, USA
* Corresponding author. 800 Walnut Street, 18th Floor, Philadelphia, PA 19107.
E-mail address: karthik.rajasekaran@pennmedicine.upenn.edu

Otolaryngol Clin N Am 57 (2024) 635–647
https://doi.org/10.1016/j.otc.2024.02.013
0030-6665/24/© 2024 Elsevier Inc. All rights reserved.

oto.theclinics.com

addressing the underlying cancer. Initial assessment must be extensive in order to understand the underlying causes of dysphagia, goals of care, and possible therapeutic options.[3,4] Recent advances have fortunately awarded more avenues of care for dysphagia, yet close attention must be paid regarding their feasibility in the context of current or previous cancer treatments like radiotherapy.[5,6] Future plans to optimize surgical techniques, chemotherapeutic regimens, radiation modalities, and immunotherapy alongside improving symptom monitoring and supportive care aim to reduce the dysphagic burden of patients with HN cancer.[3,5] Herein, we summarize the diagnosis and management of dysphagia in patients with HN cancer from initial presentation to long-term follow-up, highlighting current strengths, weaknesses, and ongoing research.

DISCUSSION
Evaluation

History
When evaluating a patient with HN cancer for dysphagia, it is critical to obtain a thorough history. Upon diagnosis, the following cancer properties should be noted: type, location, stage, previous or current treatment, therapeutic response, and history of recurrences. Particular care should be paid to the patient's treatment as surgery, radiation (ie, both total dose and date of completion), and systemic therapy all have been correlated with dysphagia.[3,5–11] A thorough medical history alongside timing and character of dysphagic symptoms should also be closely assessed to better understand the most primary cause. Use of standardized clinician and patient-based functional scales (ie, Functional Outcomes Swallowing Score [FOSS], M.D. Anderson Dysphagia Inventory [MDADI], Eating Assessment Tool [EAT-10]) is also encouraged to better characterize dysphagic symptoms; however, full discussion of these metrics will be deferred to a later section.[12]

Physical examination
A full HN examination in these patients allows the clinician to understand the extent of their cancer and objectively assess for contributing factors to their dysphagia. Cranial nerve examination can also reveal tumor-related neuromotor dysfunction that may be responsible for patient dysphagia.[13] Aside from the neoplasm itself, it is important to note treatment-related sequelae that may manifest on physical examination.[8,14] Radiated patients should be assessed for signs of tenderness or inflammation in the early stage (ie, ongoing regimen or weeks to few months after treatment) and permanently dysfunctional, nonhealing tissue or bone in the late stage (several months to years after treatment).[5,6,9,15] Systemic therapy patients should be examined for signs of mucositis, cachexia, neuromuscular impairment, and autoimmune inflammation.[10,11,16]

Imaging and additional testing
Imaging is always utilized in the workup of patients with HN cancer, but the exact modality will be dependent on each patient's neoplasm. Computed tomography (CT) with contrast and MRI are most commonly used with the former being preferred for bony involvement and the latter for soft tissue.[1,17] These studies showcase anatomic abnormalities that can help explain the cause of the dysphagia but are often insufficient alone. A variety of different swallow-specific tests can be subsequently performed with the assistance of other health care professionals. Inpatient bedside swallow challenges by nursing staff can help as an initial screening tool in the acute setting (ie, to help dictate postoperative diet regimen); however, these

assessments should always be supplemented with a clinical swallowing evaluation from a speech-language pathologist (SLP) for the long term.[18] Objective assessment by an otolaryngologist (ear, nose, and throat [ENT] physician) with flexible fiberoptic laryngoscopy alongside formal SLP evaluation with fiberoptic endoscopic evaluation of swallowing (FEES) and video fluoroscopic swallow studies (VFSS) all provide direct insight into how cancer or treatment-related adverse effects may be impairing aerodigestive anatomy, function, and synergy throughout all phases of swallowing (**Fig. 1**).[19] FEES primarily evaluates the pharyngeal phase of swallowing and partially the oral transit phase, while providing direct visualization of oropharyngeal anatomy before and after the swallow.[20] VFSS assesses dysphagia continuously throughout the oral, pharyngeal, and upper esophageal phases of swallowing under fluoroscopy.[20] Additionally, these specialized testing modalities can be used intermittently to assess patient's dysphagic symptom progression over time (ie, consistency of food and liquid tolerances, penetration/aspiration frequency, swallowing efficiency, benefit of compensatory swallowing techniques, and so forth). For example, completing a VFSS prior to radiation treatment of HN cancer is often recommended to objectively evaluate a patient's baseline swallowing function, which can then be used for comparison to subsequent examinations if dysphagia develops.

Goals

As with any patient with cancer, it is paramount to establish goals of care soon after diagnosis. The conversation should involve a multidisciplinary team (ie, ENTs, SLPs, palliative care physicians, medical and radiation oncologists, and dieticians) and be patient-centered, ensuring that patients are decisional and adequately informed about their diagnosis and possible treatment options. For patients with curable cancer who intend to pursue treatment, clinicians should weigh the patient's severity of dysphagia in the context of their therapy regimen. Essentially, if the dysphagic sequelae are uncomfortable yet tolerable, patients may opt to continue with surgery, radiation, or systemic therapy despite the possibility of it worsening their current QOL. However, frequent encounters or hospitalizations due to malnutrition, aspiration pneumonia, and so forth should warrant prompt attention and possible modification or discontinuation of responsible treatments.[10,21] For patients with incurable

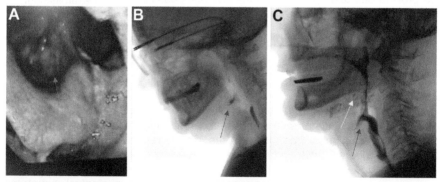

Fig. 1. Characteristic findings in dysphagic patients with HN cancer seen during (A) fiberoptic endoscopic evaluations of swallowing as well as (B, C) VFSS. The *blue arrow* points to areas of mucosal edema and inflammation along the vestibular folds status postsurgery and radiation. *Red arrows* show barium penetrating into the airway, and the yellow arrow indicates radiographic evidence of vessel clips placed intraoperatively.

cancer or those who do not wish to pursue treatment, clinicians should weigh the patient's severity of dysphagia in the context of their QOL. Notably, many patients with HN cancer consider swallowing function a primary factor regarding their QOL.[22] The definition of high QOL can vary widely among each patient with some prioritizing continuance of their activities of daily living while others valuing time and comfort at home above all else.[23,24] Therefore, the extent of dysphagia treatment should align with the patient's desired schedules with nuanced, guided counseling throughout. Additional care should still be taken to address serious complications of dysphagia, yet each patient's right to refuse treatment should also be respected.[3]

Therapeutic Options

Prevention

Prophylactic dysphagia therapy provided by SLPs prior to and concurrently during radiation treatment has proven to reduce severity of or prevent dysphagia symptoms altogether.[3,25,26] Adhering to a regular oropharyngeal swallowing exercise regimen and continuing with oral intake throughout radiation treatment improves the likelihood of maintaining a regular oral diet long-term, and consequently improving patient QOL.[22] Patients who maintain an oral diet throughout radiation treatment are twice as likely to resume normal eating following treatment than those who do not. Additionally, those who continue with oropharyngeal exercises during treatment are 4 times as likely to achieve these outcomes.[22] Though some patients may still require supplemental nutrition during treatment due to acute radiation toxicities that impact mastication and swallowing (ie, odynophagia, mucositis, dysgeusia, xerostomia, and so forth), completion of swallowing exercises throughout radiation is also associated with reduced duration of gastrostomy dependence.[22,27] These daily exercise regimens (Mendelsohn maneuver, Masako maneuver, effortful swallow, and so forth) and the continuation of oral intake throughout treatment (ie, eat all through radiation therapy) both aid in maintaining oropharyngeal muscle function and structural integrity needed to swallow efficiently and safely.[22,27-29] SLPs often guide patients through these therapies, but their success is highly dependent on patient follow through.[25,28] Counseling should therefore emphasize the importance of compliance and how patients may integrate the practices into daily routines. SLPs also provide diet texture modifications and compensatory swallowing techniques to help patients eat and drink safely after surgical resections, as well as during or following radiation treatment. On the clinician side, the use of modern cancer treatments like transoral robotic surgery, transoral laser microsurgery, and intensity-modulated radiation therapy has demonstrated improved functional swallowing outcomes relative to older modalities.[30-32]

Supportive care

Supportive care for patients with HN cancer largely depends on the characteristics of their dysphagia. Patients with xerostomia contributing to oral phase dysfunction may benefit from alcohol-free mouth rinses, dietary restrictions (ie, limit caffeine, alcohol, and sugary foods), and frequent hydration.[4,33] Odynophagia and lymphedema impairing swallow initiation can be remedied with tailored pain medication regimens and compressive therapy, respectively.[34,35] Psychological symptoms can be ameliorated by referring patients to psychiatry colleagues and HN cancer support groups.[35,36] Importantly, patient expectations should be managed by stating supportive measures provide symptomatic relief rather than definitive control.

Swallowing therapy

Swallowing therapy managed by SLPs with support from clinical dieticians has proven to be effective in treating dysphagia among patients with HN cancer.[37–40] The general principle of swallowing therapy centers around rehabilitating patients' innate swallowing function by strengthening the oropharyngeal musculature to improve oral intake and prevent aspiration.[41,42] Although implementation may vary among health care professionals, approaches commonly consist of gradual variations in mouth opening assistance to improve trismus (via physiotherapy, prosthetic devices, and so forth), bolus consistency modification, biofeedback, compensatory swallowing techniques (ie, chin down), and oropharyngeal exercise regimens or programs (ie, McNeill Dysphagia Therapy Program).[3,43] Clinicians previously championed continuation of therapy for as long as possible; however, the recent literature has called this into question, leaving ideal duration up to professional judgment.[44] Similar to prophylactic swallowing exercises, patients should be advised that their benefit is largely correlated with their adherence to recommendations.[35,45] Within the population with HN cancer, late-onset chronic dysphagia following radiation treatment is most often due to decreased strength and range of motion of the oropharyngeal musculature secondary to fibrosis, atrophy, and neuropathy, which can develop many years following treatment and is less responsive to swallowing therapy.[46] Special attention should also be paid to sarcopenic HN cancer patients. They are at especially high risk for baseline dysphagia and aspiration following radiation, so promptly diagnosing suspected patients with diminished skeletal muscle mass (ie, via CT-based calculations) could improve outcomes.[47] Therefore, patient risk stratification, preventative therapy, and early intervention from an SLP are imperative to reduce the severity of progressive radiation-induced dysphagia.

Interventional measures

A wide range of interventional measures exists to manage dysphagia in HN cancer depending on each patient's unique clinical picture. Many postoperative patients benefit from placement of a nasogastric tube—that can be later removed or transitioned to a gastrostomy tube if required after several weeks—to prevent dysphagia-related cachexia.[48] Similarly, whether necessitated by the cancer or as palliation, cuffed and uncuffed tracheostomy tubes can facilitate respiratory tract clearance to relieve aerodigestive obstructions.[49] Other treatments aimed at improving bolus transport include esophageal dilations alongside botulinum toxin injections and myotomies of the upper esophageal sphincter.[50–52] In patients with especially refractory dysphagia, depending on the tumor location and cause for dysphagia, surgeries like vocal fold augmentation, vocal fold medialization, laryngeal suspension, and even total laryngectomy can be performed.[3,53–56] The invasive nature of these procedures warrants extensive discussion with patients because although procedures can potentially improve QOL, they also have risks.

Clinical Outcomes

Monitoring functional swallow status

Per the nature of their condition, patients with HN cancer routinely return for follow-up to assess response to treatment and QOL.[35] Dysphagia can be evaluated at these visits following the previously described evaluation protocols but also can be supplemented with the variety of dysphagia scales described in **Table 1**.[57–61] Currently, no recommendations exist regarding a preferred index but several studies endorse benefits in longitudinally tracking functional statuses of patients.[62–65] As a result, it may be

Table 1
Different functional swallowing scales capable of assessing dysphagia in patients with head and neck cancer

	Name	Development Group(s)	Indication	Composition	References
Clinician-based scales	FOSS	Mayo Clinic, Jacksonville	Determination of severity of oropharyngeal dysphagia and effectiveness of therapy on outcomes	Five stages of patient stratification based on dietary modifications, nutritional status, aspiration frequency, and dysphagic symptoms	Salassa et al,[57] 2000
	Performance Status Scale for Head and Neck Cancer	University of Illinois at Chicago	Assessment of dysfunction experienced by patients with HN cancer	Twenty-one items classified within public eating, speech understandability, and diet normalcy subscales	List et al,[58] 1990
Patient-based scales	EAT-10	University of California, Davis; Medical College of Georgia	Quick evaluation of dysphagia-related symptom severity, QOL, and treatment efficacy	Ten questions on topics related to nutritional status, social impairment, and swallow function	Belafsky et al,[59] 2008
	MDADI	University of Texas M.D. Anderson Cancer Center; University of Texas School of Public Health	Assessment of impact dysphagia has on QOL in patients with HN cancer	Twenty items under global, emotional, functional, and physical domains	Chen et al,[60] 2002
	Sydney Swallow Questionnaire	St. George Hospital; University of New South Wales	Measurement of symptomatic severity of oropharyngeal dysphagia	17 questions on topics related to aspiration, swallow function, and social impairment	Wallace et al,[61] 2000

advisable for each center to uniformly adopt one clinician-based and one patient-based functional scale for use at each follow-up visit. This way values are not only consistent between each appointment but can be facilely compared between appropriate patients.

Complications, concerns, and considerations

Complications from dysphagia in HN cancer are often multifactorial. Using aspiration pneumonia as an example, the cause may be secondary to enlarging tumor mass effect, postoperative esophageal strictures, or radiation-related pharyngeal edema or fibrosis.[66–68] Similarly, malnutrition may be a result of progressive neoplastic metabolic demands, inadequately controlled odynophagia after reconstruction, or systemic therapy-induced mucositis.[69–71] It is therefore important to consider a multimodal approach when addressing these concerns. Specifically, by revisiting different therapy regimens, goals of care, and patient-specific disease courses upon presentation, clinicians can improve outcomes and QOL for dysphagic HN cancer patients.[71]

Future Directions

Ongoing research

Clinical practice guidelines (CPGs) have been developed in recent years by several professional organizations to standardize diagnosis and management of evaluation of dysphagia in HN cancer.[3,4,33,35,72] Despite their transparency regarding development, external assessments of their quality and basis in evidence-based medicine are recommended prior to widespread implementation. Regarding innovation in dysphagia evaluation methods, research is currently being done into manometry as a complement to FEES and VFSS. High-resolution manometry (HRM) provides objective data regarding the dynamics of swallowing, so advocates claim its results may be more reliable versus professional-dependent interpretation involved in VFSS; however, supporting evidence is currently sparse with no robust trials having been performed to date.[73–77] In the realm of treatment, interest in use of neuromuscular electrical stimulation (NMES) alongside traditional swallow therapy has grown significantly over the past decade.[78–84] The principle of NMES relies on repeated electrical-induced contractions progressively strengthening damaged swallowing muscles. The data advocating for its use are conflicting; older trials performed by Ryu and colleagues[81] and Long and colleagues[84] showed benefit of NMES relative to isolated swallow therapy while a newer, larger trial performed by Langmore and colleagues[78] found no significant difference. Given the invasive nature of NMES, caution regarding implementation should be exercised until additional data are released.

SUMMARY

Overall, diagnosis and management of dysphagia in patients with HN cancer is a dynamic process that involves continued consideration throughout their course of disease. Initial evaluation should provide comprehensive information about their neoplasm and associated treatments via history taking, physical examination, and dysphagia-specific imaging. Their goals of care should be obtained and weighed during choice of therapy. Prevention is a valuable form of treatment which should later be supplemented by supportive care, swallowing therapy, and interventional measures when indicated. Referral to an SLP prior to radiation for prophylactic intervention can help improve dysphagia outcomes following treatment. Response and necessary modifications to treatment should be closely monitored via standardized functional scales and reported complications. Finally, close attention should be paid to new CPGs and how HRM and NMES will influence the future of care for patients with HN cancer.

CLINICS CARE POINTS

- Workup for dysphagia in patients with HN cancer requires additional, specific imaging such as FEES and VFSS
- Patient wishes to not pursue care must be respected
- Prophylactic swallowing therapy and continued oral intake during radiation treatment can improve dysphagia
- Counseling should emphasize the importance of patient compliance regarding dysphagia therapies and risk of late-onset radiation-induced dysphagia
- No gold standard of outcome monitoring exists; consistency and prompt, appropriate modification of treatment regimens are more important
- Await further research before fully implementing CPGs, HRM, and NMES into clinical practice for dysphagic patients with HN cancer

DISCLOSURE

The authors have no conflicts of interest to disclose. No funding was received for conducting this study.

REFERENCES

1. National Comprehensive Cancer Network. Head and Neck Cancers (Version 1.2024). Available at: https://www.nccn.org/professionals/physician_gls/pdf/head-and-neck.pdf. [Accessed 16 November 2023].
2. Krebbers I, Pilz W, Vanbelle S, et al. Affective Symptoms and Oropharyngeal Dysphagia in Head-and-Neck Cancer Patients: A Systematic Review. Dysphagia 2023;38(1):127–44.
3. Baijens LWJ, Walshe M, Aaltonen LM, et al. European white paper: oropharyngeal dysphagia in head and neck cancer. Eur Arch Oto-Rhino-Laryngol 2021;278(2):577–616.
4. Cohen EEW, LaMonte SJ, Erb NL, et al. American Cancer Society Head and Neck Cancer Survivorship Care Guideline. CA A Cancer J Clin 2016;66(3):203–39.
5. Greco E, Simic T, Ringash J, et al. Dysphagia Treatment for Patients With Head and Neck Cancer Undergoing Radiation Therapy: A Meta-analysis Review. Int J Radiat Oncol Biol Phys 2018;101(2):421–44.
6. Strojan P, Hutcheson KA, Eisbruch A, et al. Treatment of late sequelae after radiotherapy for head and neck cancer. Cancer Treat Rev 2017;59:79–92.
7. Pezdirec M, Strojan P, Boltezar IH. Swallowing disorders after treatment for head and neck cancer. Radiol Oncol 2019;53(2):225–30.
8. Kronenberger MB, Meyers AD. Dysphagia following head and neck cancer surgery. Dysphagia 1994;9(4):236–44.
9. Brook I. Early side effects of radiation treatment for head and neck cancer. Cancer Radiother 2021;25(5):507–13.

10. Denaro N, Merlano MC, Russi EG. Dysphagia in Head and Neck Cancer Patients: Pretreatment Evaluation, Predictive Factors, and Assessment during Radio-Chemotherapy, Recommendations. Clin Exp Otorhinolaryngol 2013;6(3):117.

11. Moroney LB, Helios J, Ward EC, et al. Patterns of dysphagia and acute toxicities in patients with head and neck cancer undergoing helical IMRT±concurrent chemotherapy. Oral Oncol 2017;64:1–8.

12. Yao CMKL, Hutcheson KA. Quality of Life Implications After Transoral Robotic Surgery for Oropharyngeal Cancers. Otolaryngol Clin 2020;53(6):1117–29.

13. Carter RL, Pittam MR, Tanner NSB. Pain and Dysphagia in Patients with Squamous Carcinomas of the Head and Neck: The Role of Perineural Spread. J R Soc Med 1982;75(8):598–606.

14. Manikantan K, Khode S, Sayed SI, et al. Dysphagia in head and neck cancer. Cancer Treat Rev 2009;35(8):724–32.

15. King SN, Dunlap NE, Tennant PA, et al. Pathophysiology of Radiation-Induced Dysphagia in Head and Neck Cancer. Dysphagia 2016;31(3):339–51.

16. Wang H, Mustafa A, Liu S, et al. Immune Checkpoint Inhibitor Toxicity in Head and Neck Cancer: From Identification to Management. Front Pharmacol 2019; 10:1254.

17. Mesia R, Iglesias L, Lambea J, et al. SEOM clinical guidelines for the treatment of head and neck cancer (2020). Clin Transl Oncol 2021;23(5):913–21.

18. Bours GJJW, Speyer R, Lemmens J, et al. Bedside screening tests vs. videofluoroscopy or fibreoptic endoscopic evaluation of swallowing to detect dysphagia in patients with neurological disorders: systematic review. J Adv Nurs 2009;65(3): 477–93.

19. Denk-Linnert DM, Farneti D, Nawka T, et al. Position Statement of the Union of European Phoniatricians (UEP): Fees and Phoniatricians' Role in Multidisciplinary and Multiprofessional Dysphagia Management Team. Dysphagia 2023;38(2): 711–8.

20. Giraldo-Cadavid LF, Leal-Leaño LR, Leon-Basantes GA, et al. Accuracy of endoscopic and videofluoroscopic evaluations of swallowing for oropharyngeal dysphagia. Laryngoscope 2017;127(9):2002–10.

21. Gaziano JE. Evaluation and Management of Oropharyngeal Dysphagia in Head and Neck Cancer. Cancer Control 2002;9(5):400–9.

22. Hutcheson KA, Bhayani MK, Beadle BM, et al. Eat and Exercise During Radiotherapy or Chemoradiotherapy for Pharyngeal Cancers: Use It or Lose It. JAMA Otolaryngol Head Neck Surg 2013;139(11):1127.

23. Carr AJ. Measuring quality of life: Is quality of life determined by expectations or experience? BMJ 2001;322(7296):1240–3.

24. Shrestha A, Martin C, Burton M, et al. Quality of life versus length of life considerations in cancer patients: A systematic literature review. Psycho Oncol 2019; 28(7):1367–80.

25. Loewen I, Jeffery CC, Rieger J, et al. Prehabilitation in head and neck cancer patients: a literature review. J of Otolaryngol - Head & Neck Surg. 2021;50(1):2.

26. Kotz T, Federman AD, Kao J, et al. Prophylactic Swallowing Exercises in Patients With Head and Neck Cancer Undergoing Chemoradiation. Arch Otolaryngol Head Neck Surg 2012;138(4).

27. Hutcheson KA, Gomes A, Rodriguez V, et al. Eat All Through Radiation Therapy (EAT-RT): Structured therapy model to facilitate continued oral intake through head and neck radiotherapy—User acceptance and content validation. Head Neck 2020;42(9):2390–6.

28. Starmer HM. Dysphagia in head and neck cancer: prevention and treatment. Curr Opin Otolaryngol Head Neck Surg 2014;22(3):195–200.
29. Langmore S, Krisciunas GP, Miloro KV, et al. Does PEG Use Cause Dysphagia in Head and Neck Cancer Patients? Dysphagia 2012;27(2):251–9.
30. Iseli TA, Kulbersh BD, Iseli CE, et al. Functional Outcomes after Transoral Robotic Surgery for Head and Neck Cancer. Otolaryngol Head Neck Surg 2009;141(2): 166–71.
31. Nasef HO, Thabet H, Piazza C, et al. Prospective analysis of functional swallowing outcome after resection of T2 glottic carcinoma using transoral laser surgery and external vertical hemilaryngectomy. Eur Arch Oto-Rhino-Laryngol 2016; 273(8):2133–40.
32. Nutting C, Finneran L, Roe J, et al. Dysphagia-optimised intensity-modulated radiotherapy versus standard intensity-modulated radiotherapy in patients with head and neck cancer (DARS): a phase 3, multicentre, randomised, controlled trial. Lancet Oncol 2023;24(8):868–80.
33. Verdonck-de Leeuw I, Dawson C, Licitra L, et al. European Head and Neck Society recommendations for head and neck cancer survivorship care. Oral Oncol 2022;133:106047.
34. Bossi P, Giusti R, Tarsitano A, et al. The point of pain in head and neck cancer. Crit Rev Oncol Hematol 2019;138:51–9.
35. Goyal N, Day A, Epstein J, et al. Head and neck cancer survivorship consensus statement from the American Head and Neck Society. Laryngoscope Investig Oto 2022;7(1):70–92.
36. Murphy BA, Deng J. Advances in Supportive Care for Late Effects of Head and Neck Cancer. J Clin Orthod 2015;33(29):3314–21.
37. Talwar B, Donnelly R, Skelly R, et al. Nutritional management in head and neck cancer: United Kingdom National Multidisciplinary Guidelines. J Laryngol Otol 2016;130(S2):S32–40.
38. Kristensen MB, Isenring E, Brown B. Nutrition and swallowing therapy strategies for patients with head and neck cancer. Nutrition 2020;69:110548.
39. Banda KJ, Chu H, Kao CC, et al. Swallowing exercises for head and neck cancer patients: A systematic review and meta-analysis of randomized control trials. Int J Nurs Stud 2021;114:103827.
40. Rodriguez AM, Komar A, Ringash J, et al. A scoping review of rehabilitation interventions for survivors of head and neck cancer. Disabil Rehabil 2019;41(17): 2093–107.
41. Owen S, Paleri V. Laryngectomy rehabilitation in the United Kingdom. Curr Opin Otolaryngol Head Neck Surg 2013;21(3):186–91.
42. Hajdú SF, Wessel I, Dalton SO, et al. Swallowing Exercise During Head and Neck Cancer Treatment: Results of a Randomized Trial. Dysphagia 2022;37(4):749–62.
43. Crary MA, Carnaby GD, LaGorio LA, et al. Functional and Physiological Outcomes from an Exercise-Based Dysphagia Therapy: A Pilot Investigation of the McNeill Dysphagia Therapy Program. Arch Phys Med Rehabil 2012;93(7): 1173–8.
44. Langmore SE, Pisegna JM. Efficacy of exercises to rehabilitate dysphagia: A critique of the literature. Int J Speech Lang Pathol 2015;17(3):222–9.
45. Kamstra JI, Van Leeuwen M, Roodenburg JLN, et al. Exercise therapy for trismus secondary to head and neck cancer: A systematic review. Head Neck 2017; 39(1):160–9.
46. Hutcheson KA, Lewin JS, Barringer DA, et al. Late dysphagia after radiotherapy-based treatment of head and neck cancer. Cancer 2012;118(23):5793–9.

47. Colback AA, Arkfeld DV, Evangelista LM, et al. Effect of Sarcopenia on Swallowing in Patients With Head and Neck Cancer. Otolaryngology-Head Neck Surg (Tokyo) 2024. https://doi.org/10.1002/ohn.655. n/a(n/a).

48. Wang J, Liu M, Liu C, et al. Percutaneous endoscopic gastrostomy versus nasogastric tube feeding for patients with head and neck cancer: a systematic review. J Radiat Res 2014;55(3):559–67.

49. Skoretz SA, Anger N, Wellman L, et al. A Systematic Review of Tracheostomy Modifications and Swallowing in Adults. Dysphagia 2020;35(6):935–47.

50. Moss WJ, Pang J, Orosco RK, et al. Esophageal dilation in head and neck cancer patients: A systematic review and meta-analysis. Laryngoscope 2018;128(1): 111–7.

51. Lightbody K, Wilkie M, Kinshuck A, et al. Injection of botulinum toxin for the treatment of post-laryngectomy pharyngoesophageal spasm-related disorders. Annals 2015;97(7):508–12.

52. Kocdor P, Siegel ER, Tulunay-Ugur OE. Cricopharyngeal dysfunction: A systematic review comparing outcomes of dilatation, botulinum toxin injection, and myotomy. Laryngoscope 2016;126(1):135–41.

53. Dion GR, Nielsen SW. In-Office Laryngology Injections. Otolaryngol Clin 2019; 52(3):521–36.

54. Barbu AM, Gniady JP, Vivero RJ, et al. Bedside Injection Medialization Laryngoplasty in Immediate Postoperative Patients. Otolaryngol Head Neck Surg 2015; 153(6):1007–12.

55. Fujimoto Y, Hasegawa Y, Yamada H, et al. Swallowing Function Following Extensive Resection of Oral or Oropharyngeal Cancer With Laryngeal Suspension and Cricopharyngeal Myotomy. Laryngoscope 2007;117(8):1343–8.

56. Hutcheson KA, Alvarez CP, Barringer DA, et al. Outcomes of Elective Total Laryngectomy for Laryngopharyngeal Dysfunction in Disease-Free Head and Neck Cancer Survivors. Otolaryngol Head Neck Surg 2012;146(4):585–90.

57. Salassa J. A Functional Outcome Swallowing Scale for Staging Oropharyngeal Dysphagia. Dig Dis 2000;17(4):230–4.

58. List MA, Ritter-Sterr C, Lansky SB. A performance status scale for head and neck cancer patients. Cancer 1990;66(3):564–9.

59. Belafsky PC, Mouadeb DA, Rees CJ, et al. Validity and Reliability of the Eating Assessment Tool (EAT-10). Ann Otol Rhinol Laryngol 2008;117(12):919–24.

60. Chen AY, Frankowski R, Bishop-Leone J, et al. The Development and Validation of a Dysphagia-Specific Quality-of-Life Questionnaire for Patients With Head and Neck Cancer: The M. D. Anderson Dysphagia Inventory. Arch Otolaryngol Head Neck Surg 2001;127(7):870–6.

61. Wallace KL, Middleton S, Cook IJ. Development and validation of a self-report symptom inventory to assess the severity of oral-pharyngeal dysphagia. Gastroenterology 2000;118(4):678–87.

62. Goepfert RP, Lewin JS, Barrow MP, et al. Long-Term, Prospective Performance of the MD Anderson Dysphagia Inventory in "Low-Intermediate Risk" Oropharyngeal Carcinoma After Intensity Modulated Radiation Therapy. Int J Radiat Oncol Biol Phys 2017;97(4):700–8.

63. Høxbroe Michaelsen S, Grønhøj C, Høxbroe Michaelsen J, et al. Quality of life in survivors of oropharyngeal cancer: A systematic review and meta-analysis of 1366 patients. Eur J Cancer 2017;78:91–102.

64. Starmer HM, Klein D, Montgomery A, et al. Head and Neck Virtual Coach: A Randomized Control Trial of Mobile Health as an Adjunct to Swallowing Therapy During Head and Neck Radiation. Dysphagia 2023;38(3):847–55.

65. Sinn FS, Charters E, Stone D, et al. Responsiveness of the EAT-10 to Clinical Change in Head and Neck Cancer Patients with Dysphagia. Int J Speech Lang Pathol 2020;22(1):78–85.

66. Funakawa K, Uto H, Sasaki F, et al. Effect of Endoscopic Submucosal Dissection for Superficial Esophageal Neoplasms and Risk Factors for Postoperative Stricture. Medicine 2015;94(1):e373.

67. Francis DO, Weymuller EA, Parvathaneni U, et al. Dysphagia, Stricture, and Pneumonia in Head and Neck Cancer Patients: Does Treatment Modality Matter? Ann Otol Rhinol Laryngol 2010;119(6):391–7.

68. Jakobi A, Bandurska-Luque A, Stützer K, et al. Identification of Patient Benefit From Proton Therapy for Advanced Head and Neck Cancer Patients Based on Individual and Subgroup Normal Tissue Complication Probability Analysis. Int J Radiat Oncol Biol Phys 2015;92(5):1165–74.

69. Thambamroong T, Seetalarom K, Saichaemchan S, et al. Efficacy of Curcumin on Treating Cancer Anorexia-Cachexia Syndrome in Locally or Advanced Head and Neck Cancer: A Double-Blind, Placebo-Controlled Randomised Phase IIa Trial (CurChexia). In: Gumpricht E, editor. Journal of Nutrition and Metabolism 2022; 2022:1–11.

70. Parke SC, Langelier DM, Cheng JT, et al. State of Rehabilitation Research in the Head and Neck Cancer Population: Functional Impact vs. Impairment-Focused Outcomes. Curr Oncol Rep 2022;24(4):517–32.

71. Crowder SL, Douglas KG, Yanina Pepino M, et al. Nutrition impact symptoms and associated outcomes in post-chemoradiotherapy head and neck cancer survivors: a systematic review. J Cancer Surviv 2018;12(4):479–94.

72. Clarke P, Radford K, Coffey M, et al. Speech and swallow rehabilitation in head and neck cancer: United Kingdom National Multidisciplinary Guidelines. J Laryngol Otol 2016;130(S2):S176–80.

73. Szczesniak MM, Maclean J, Zhang T, et al. Inter-rater reliability and validity of automated impedance manometry analysis and fluoroscopy in dysphagic patients after head and neck cancer radiotherapy. Neurogastroenterology Motil 2015;27(8):1183–9.

74. Schar MS, Omari TI, Woods CM, et al. Pharyngeal tongue base augmentation for dysphagia therapy: A prospective case series in patients post head and neck cancer treatment. Head Neck 2022;44(8):1871–84.

75. Schaen-Heacock NE, Jones CA, McCulloch TM. Pharyngeal Swallowing Pressures in Patients with Radiation-Associated Dysphagia. Dysphagia 2021;36(2): 242–9.

76. Pauloski BR, Rademaker AW, Lazarus C, et al. Relationship Between Manometric and Videofluoroscopic Measures of Swallow Function in Healthy Adults and Patients Treated for Head and Neck Cancer with Various Modalities. Dysphagia 2009;24(2):196–203.

77. Lenius K, Stierwalt J, LaPointe LL, et al. Effects of Lingual Effort on Swallow Pressures Following Radiation Treatment. J Speech Lang Hear Res 2015;58(3): 687–97.

78. Langmore SE, McCulloch TM, Krisciunas GP, et al. Efficacy of electrical stimulation and exercise for dysphagia in patients with head and neck cancer: A randomized clinical trial. Head Neck 2016;38(S1).

79. Peng G, Masood K, Gantz O, et al. Neuromuscular electrical stimulation improves radiation-induced fibrosis through Tgf-B1/MyoD homeostasis in head and neck cancer. J Surg Oncol 2016;114(1):27–31.

80. Bhatt AD, Goodwin N, Cash E, et al. Impact of transcutaneous neuromuscular electrical stimulation on dysphagia in patients with head and neck cancer treated with definitive chemoradiation. Head Neck 2015;37(7):1051–6.
81. Ryu JS, Kang JY, Park JY, et al. The effect of electrical stimulation therapy on dysphagia following treatment for head and neck cancer. Oral Oncol 2009; 45(8):665–8.
82. Costa DR, Santos PSDS, Fischer Rubira CM, et al. Immediate effect of neuromuscular electrical stimulation on swallowing function in individuals after oral and oropharyngeal cancer therapy. SAGE Open Medicine 2020;8. 2050312120 97415.
83. Van Daele DJ, Langmore SE, Krisciunas GP, et al. The impact of time after radiation treatment on dysphagia in patients with head and neck cancer enrolled in a swallowing therapy program. Head Neck 2019;41(3):606–14.
84. Long YB, Wu XP. A randomized controlled trial of combination therapy of neuromuscular electrical stimulation and balloon dilatation in the treatment of radiation-induced dysphagia in nasopharyngeal carcinoma patients. Disabil Rehabil 2013; 35(6):450–4.

Tracheostomy-Related Swallowing Issues in Children

Eileen M. Raynor, MD[a],*, Daniel Wohl, MD[b,1]

KEYWORDS

- Pediatric tracheostomy • Dysphagia • PMV • Decannulation • Aspiration
- Tracheostomy tube

KEY POINTS

- Children with tracheostomies have prolonged swallowing time and restriction of laryngeal motion during swallows.
- Alteration in sensitivity in the upper aerodigestive tract due to intubation or tracheostomy may contribute to worse oropharyngeal dysphagia in these children.
- The use of Passy Muir valve or capping improves swallow function and may decrease aspiration.
- Pediatric feeding disorders may accompany oropharyngeal dysphagia in tracheostomy extending time needed to attain oral feeding.

BACKGROUND

With improvement in critical care management of children and infants, there is a higher incidence of prolonged orotracheal intubation as well as tracheostomy placement. Evidence has shown that these children have a significantly higher risk of need for alimentary nutrition via nasogastric or gastrostomy tubes and are prone to develop moderate-to-severe oropharyngeal dysphagia as well as other pediatric feeding disorders like oral aversion.[1–3] The incidence of postextubation dysphagia ranges from 30% to 84%, though fortunately a majority of this is temporary in nature.[2–4]

Children who undergo tracheostomy, do so for a variety of conditions ranging from upper airway obstruction, chronic lung disease to neurologic deficits. Children with underlying neurologic, gastrointestinal, or cardiac conditions are predisposed to dysphagia independent of having a tracheostomy.[5,6] Ventilator-dependent children

[a] Department of Head and Neck Surgery & Communication Sciences, Duke Health System, DUMC Box 3805, Durham, NC 27710, USA; [b] Pediatric Otolaryngology Associates, 4114 Sunbeam Road, Jacksonville, FL 32257, USA
[1] Present address: 9003 Kings Colony Road, Jacksonville, FL 32257.
* Corresponding author. 2212 Timberview Drive, Durham, NC 27705.
E-mail address: Eileen.raynor@duke.edu

Otolaryngol Clin N Am 57 (2024) 649–655
https://doi.org/10.1016/j.otc.2024.02.017
0030-6665/24/© 2024 Elsevier Inc. All rights reserved.

with tracheostomies are particularly vulnerable to dysphagia due to the need for an unoccluded, possibly cuffed tracheostomy tube as well as movement from the ventilator circuit.[7]

IMPACT ON SWALLOW

Normal swallowing requires a sequence of events in the oral cavity, oropharynx, and pharynx to achieve adequate deglutition and prevention of aspiration. **Box 1** shows the components of a normal swallowing mechanism.[8] Swallowing is characterized by phases: the preoral preparatory phase involving olfaction, cognition, and visual inputs. Next is the oral phase where food is introduced into the mouth, and the tongue and facial muscles form a bolus and propel it toward the pharynx. The pharyngeal phase includes the laryngeal and pharyngeal sensory receptors to trigger laryngeal activity and allow for opening of the upper esophageal sphincter. Finally, the esophageal phase occurs when the bolus passes beyond the upper esophageal sphincter.[8]

The presence of a tracheostomy impacts swallow mechanics in several ways. There is a restriction in laryngeal elevation and closure of the arytenoids as well as diminished sensation in the upper airway leading to high risk of aspiration. It has been estimated that almost 95% of children with tracheostomy have evidence of aspiration with over 50% of those having silent aspiration.[9] This can lead to chronic lung disease and further dependence on the tracheostomy for adequate ventilation and oxygenation. **Fig. 1** shows a sagittal computerized tomography scan (CT) demonstrating the impact of the tracheostomy tube on the upper airway.

Oral Transit and Laryngeal Elevation

Children with tracheostomies have delays in oral transit, laryngeal vestibule closure, pharyngeal swallow initiation, and cricopharyngeal opening.[10–13] One study on adults demonstrated the odds of aspiration were twice as high with an open trach tube than with a closed (valve or cap) tube.[14] Another study demonstrated improvement when using the speaking valve and expiration.[15]

Children who can tolerate use of the Passy Muir valve (PMV) did not seem to demonstrate less aspiration, although there was less residue in the pyriform sinus seen by videofluoroscopic swallow study (VFSS) primarily with purees over thin liquids.[16] Other

---

Box 1
Components of pharyngeal swallow

- Closure of velopharyngeal port
- Elevation and anterior movement of the hyoid and larynx
- Closure of the larynx and laryngeal vestibule
  - True vocal fold adduction and cessation of respiration
  - False vocal fold contraction
  - Arytenoids tilt forward to contact the epiglottic base
  - Epiglottic inversion
- Opening of the cricopharyngeal sphincter
- Base of tongue retraction/pharyngeal wall contraction
- Progressive top-to-bottom contraction in the pharyngeal constrictors

Courtesy of Passy-Muir, Inc. Irvine, CA.

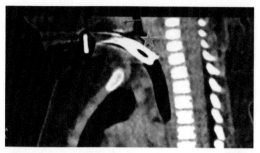

Fig. 1. Sagittal CT image of upper airway and tracheostomy showing relationship to laryngeal structures and esophagus. Red arrow: base of tongue; blue star: upper airway above the trach tube.

studies showed improvement with the use of PMV or capping due to improved laryngeal sensation and restoration of subglottic air pressure.[11,17,18]

Subglottic Pressure

One important factor in swallowing is the ability to generate subglottic pressure in order to engage laryngeal movement, glottic closure, and opening of the upper esophageal sphincter. Subglottic pressure also provides the ability to cough when food or liquid inadvertently enters the airway. Tracheostomy tubes bypass the upper airway, and therefore, the patient cannot generate adequate subglottic pressure, leading to an ineffective cough mechanism that would normally clear debris from the airway.[9,16,19] The lack of subglottic pressure has also been attributed to a greater depth of laryngeal penetration, longer bolus transit times, as well as longer pharyngeal muscle contraction.[14,17,18]

IMPACT OF CUFFED TRACHEOSTOMY TUBES

Cuffed tracheostomy tubes initially were thought to be protective of aspiration; however, recent studies have shown increased risk of aspiration due to body movement or manipulation of the tracheostomy tube with the cuff inflated.[7,11,17] Restriction of laryngeal elevation due to an inflated cuff is felt to be one reason for the increased risk of aspiration in this setting. Cuff deflation is necessary for the use of a PMV or cap to allow for laryngeal respiration and improvement in conditions necessary for effective swallowing.[11,17,20,21]

SWALLOWING ASSESSMENT IN TRACHEOSTOMY

Swallowing assessment is covered in a previous chapter (see Eileen Raynor and Jennifer Kern article, "Assessing Dysphagia in the Child," in this issue.), but in children with tracheostomy, the addition of the modified Evans blue dye test can be performed as a screening tool for aspiration. This involves placing a small amount of blue dye mixed with food or liquid on the tongue and assessing for evidence of blue-tinged secretions within the tracheostomy tube. This can be done prior to more formal instrumented assessments of swallow.[4,11,22–24] Both VFSS and flexible fiberoptic endoscopic evaluation of swallowing (FEES) are used to demonstrate the presence of aspiration and penetration with VFSS also being able to visualize the tracheostomy and presence of aspirated contents to the level of the tracheostomy tube.[24,25] Another study utilizing VFSS demonstrated a high number of children particularly in the under

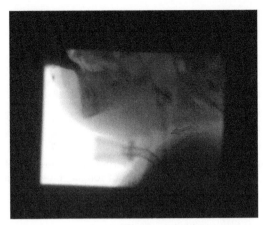

Fig. 2. A VFSS with tracheostomy and no evidence of aspiration. Red arrow: barium column.

3 year age range had significant gastroesophageal reflux which can affect efficacy of swallow or cause secondary aspiration of refluxate.[11,12] Several researchers recommend performing the swallow study in the open and occluded states to identify other causes of dysphagia in addition to the tracheostomy tube.[15,17,26,27] **Fig. 2** shows a VFSS with an occluded trach and no evidence of aspiration.

OTHER FEEDING ISSUES

Pediatric feeding disorders are also commonly seen in children with tracheostomies due to lack of oral feeding when orotracheally intubated, concern for aspiration, or difficulty with feeding therapy. These include oral refusal or aversion, spitting out of oral contents, or delayed swallowing. Several studies have shown a link between length of orotracheal intubation and pediatric feeding disorders; however, younger age at tracheostomy and lack of oral feeding from age 0 to 24 months are also risk factors.[1,4,5,28] Engagement with speech-language pathologists (SLPs) in the multidisciplinary management of these children can allow for transition to oral feeding over time. These professionals need to be engaged as soon as possible for children with tracheostomies to maximize their potential for oral feeding and actively engage with the care team on the safest way to progress toward oral feeding.[5,10,11]

DECANNULATION

Tracheostomy decannulation is what all families of children with tracheostomies hope for, this not only allows for better vocalization, ability to be safe around water but can also accelerate the progress toward oral feeding. A study of 13 children by Kang and colleagues did not show improvement in dysphagia upon decannulation when comparing VFSS in capped tracheostomy versus decannulation state[29]; however, several other studies including one by Mah and colleagues on over 300 patients showed significant improvement in swallow upon decannulation especially when a multidisciplinary team consisting of an SLP familiar with tracheostomy feeding was involved.[30,31]

SUMMARY

Children with tracheostomies have complex medical needs that may contribute independently to dysphagia and prevent transition to becoming fully oral feeders.

The involvement of a feeding specialist (SLP) in the care of these children is important to assess for dysphagia and the presence of a pediatric feeding disorder. These children are at high risk for aspiration due to the elimination of subglottic pressure and alteration of swallowing mechanics from the presence of the tracheostomy tube. Children should be assessed for ability to use a PMV or cap which can therefore enhance the oropharyngeal swallow mechanism and decrease the risk of aspiration. Instrumented swallow studies such as VFSS or FEES provide valuable information to the feeding therapist and family about the safety of different consistencies and the amounts that the child can take orally. Continued assessments while the child has the tracheostomy in place are important to determine ability to progress to more oral feeding or whether there has been any deterioration in the swallow function.

CLINICS CARE POINTS

- Children with tracheostomies often have multiple reasons for dysphagia and require a team approach to determine safety of oral feeding.
- The use of tracheostomy occlusion devices such as PMV or capping can facilitate better swallowing and allow for therapeutic progress in feeding.
- Younger children (under the age of 2 years) who have had tracheostomies for most of their life are likely to also have pediatric feeding disorders that impact their ability to eat orally.
- Multidisciplinary management and early involvement of an SLP skilled in tracheostomy care is vital for successful transition to oral feeding.
- Periodic reassessment is important to determine the status of swallowing mechanism and continued safety of oral feeding.

DISCLOSURE

The author has no relevant disclosures.

REFERENCES

1. Goday PS, Huh SY, Silverman A, et al. Pediatric feeding disorder: consensus definition and conceptual framework. J Pediatr Gastroenterol Nutr 2019;68(1):124–9.
2. Hoffmeister J, Zaborek N, Thibeault SL. Postextubation dysphagia in pediatric populations: incidence, risk factors, and outcomes. J Pediatr 2019;211:126–33. e1.
3. Horton J, Atwood C, Gnagi S, et al. Temporal trends of pediatric dysphagia in hospitalized patients. Dysphagia 2018;33:655–61.
4. Melo CCd, Paniagua LM, Signorini AV, et al. Swallowing and feeding outcomes associated with orotracheal intubation and tracheostomy in pediatrics. Audiology-Communication Research 2022;27.
5. Sharp WG, Volkert VM, Scahill L, et al. A systematic review and meta-analysis of intensive multidisciplinary intervention for pediatric feeding disorders: how standard is the standard of care? J Pediatr 2017;181:116–24. e4.
6. Skoretz SA, Anger N, Wellman L, et al. A systematic review of tracheostomy modifications and swallowing in adults. Dysphagia 2020;35:935–47.
7. Leder SB, Baker KE, Goodman TR. Dysphagia testing and aspiration status in medically stable infants requiring mechanical ventilation via tracheotomy. Pediatr Crit Care Med 2010;11(4):484–7.

8. Bartow C, King K. Impact of a tracheostomy on swallowing. Dysphagia Café; 2020.

9. Streppel M, Veder LL, Pullens B, et al. Swallowing problems in children with a tracheostomy tube. Int J Pediatr Otorhinolaryngol 2019;124:30–3.

10. Abraham SS, Wolf EL. Swallowing physiology of toddlers with long-term tracheostomies: a preliminary study. Dysphagia 2000;15:206–12.

11. Bailey RL. Tracheostomy and dysphagia: A complex association. Perspectives on Swallowing and Swallowing Disorders (Dysphagia) 2005;14(4):2–7.

12. Norman V, Louw B, Kritzinger A. Incidence and description of dysphagia in infants and toddlers with tracheostomies: A retrospective review. Int J Pediatr Otorhinolaryngol 2007;71(7):1087–92.

13. Luu K, Belsky MA, Dharmarajan H, et al. Dysphagia in pediatric patients with tracheostomy. Ann Otol Rhinol Laryngol 2022;131(5):457–62.

14. Marvin S, Thibeault SL. Predictors of aspiration and silent aspiration in patients with new tracheostomy. Am J Speech Lang Pathol 2021;30(6):2554–60.

15. Prigent H, Lejaille M, Terzi N, et al. Effect of a tracheostomy speaking valve on breathing–swallowing interaction. Intensive Care Med 2012;38:85–90.

16. Ongkasuwan J, Turk CL, Rappazzo CA, et al. The effect of a speaking valve on laryngeal aspiration and penetration in children with tracheotomies. Laryngoscope 2014;124(6):1469–74 (In eng).

17. Suiter DM, McCullough GH, Powell PW. Effects of cuff deflation and one-way tracheostomy speaking valve placement on swallow physiology. Dysphagia 2003; 18:284–92.

18. Zabih W, Holler T, Syed F, et al. The use of speaking valves in children with tracheostomy tubes. Respir Care 2017;62(12):1594–601.

19. Gross RD, Carrau RL, Slivka WA, et al. Deglutitive subglottic air pressure and respiratory system recoil. Dysphagia 2012;27:452–9.

20. Leder SB, Tarro JM, Burrell MI. Effect of occlusion of a tracheotomy tube on aspiration. Dysphagia 1996;11:254–8.

21. Rosenbek JC, Robbins JA, Roecker EB, et al. A penetration-aspiration scale. Dysphagia 1996;11:93–8.

22. Donzelli J, Brady S, Wesling M, et al. Secretions, occlusion status, and swallowing in patients with a tracheotomy tube: a descriptive study. Ear Nose Throat J 2006;85(12):831–4.

23. Cameron J, Reynolds J, Zuidema G. Aspiration in patients with tracheostomies. Surg Gynecol Obstet 1973;136(1):68–70.

24. Ceriana P, Carlucci A, Schreiber A, et al. Changes of swallowing function after tracheostomy: a videofluoroscopy study. Minerva Anestesiol 2015;81(4):389–97.

25. Tutor JD, Gosa MM. Dysphagia and aspiration in children. Pediatr Pulmonol 2012; 47(4):321–37.

26. Gross RD, Mahlmann J, Grayhack JP. Physiologic effects of open and closed tracheostomy tubes on the pharyngeal swallow. Ann Otol Rhinol Laryngol 2003; 112(2):143–52.

27. O'Connor LR, Morris NR, Paratz J. Physiological and clinical outcomes associated with use of one-way speaking valves on tracheostomised patients: A systematic review. Heart Lung 2019;48(4):356–64.

28. Henningfeld J, Lang C, Erato G, et al. Feeding disorders in children with tracheostomy tubes. Nutr Clin Pract 2021;36(3):689–95.

29. Kang JY, Choi KH, Yun GJ, et al. Does removal of tracheostomy affect dysphagia? A kinematic analysis. Dysphagia 2012;27:498–503.

30. Jung SJ, Kim DY, Kim YW, et al. Effect of decannulation on pharyngeal and laryn-geal movement in post-stroke tracheostomized patients. Annals of Rehabilitation Medicine 2012;36(3):356–64.
31. Mah JW, Staff II, Fisher SR, et al. Improving decannulation and swallowing func-tion: a comprehensive, multidisciplinary approach to post-tracheostomy care. Respir Care 2017;137–43.

Dysphagia as a Manifestation of Endocrine and Metabolic Disorders

Chloe Santa Maria, MD, MPH, Karla O'Dell, MD*

KEYWORDS

- Dysphagia • Metabolic disease • Systemic disease • Endocrine disorders
- Esophageal dysmotility • Myopathy • Neuropathy

KEY POINTS

- Dysphagia is a common manifestation of different metabolic diseases.
- Chronic hyperglycemia can result in neuropathy which produces esophageal dysmotility and gastroparesis, which can present as solid food dysphagia and slow swallowing.
- Other endocrine conditions and electrolyte disorders can cause alterations in neuromuscular excitability, which can manifest as swallowing muscular weakness, muscular spasm, and/or motility disorders.
- External compression of the pharynx in the form of a thyroid goiter, enlarged parathyroid adenoma, or cervical osteophyte also contributes to swallowing difficulty.

INTRODUCTION

Swallowing is a complex neuromuscular process, with an interplay of sensation, motor control, and coordination. There are voluntary and involuntary aspects of swallowing with control from central, peripheral somatic, and autonomic nervous systems. There needs to be a precise timed order of muscular movements starting in the oral cavity, oropharynx, laryngopharynx, and esophagus. Disruptions in any of these areas can cause significant dysphagia. Endocrine and metabolic disorders are systemic conditions with effects on whole body systems. As such, dysphagia is a common manifestation of endocrine and metabolic diseases. They can cause neuropathies and myopathies that affect the fine muscular control and coordination required for swallowing. Chronic dysphagia can lead to malnutrition; however, malnutrition particularly in the context of critical illness can independently cause pharyngeal muscle atrophy, worsen deconditioning, and produce significant dysphagia. The exact prevalence of underlying metabolic disorders in patients with dysphagia is hard to estimate as

Caruso Department of Otolaryngology Head & Neck Surgery, USC Voice Center, University of Southern California, 1537 Norfolk Street, Suite 5800, Los Angeles, CA 90033, USA
* Corresponding author.
E-mail address: karla.odell@med.usc.edu

Otolaryngol Clin N Am 57 (2024) 657–668
https://doi.org/10.1016/j.otc.2024.02.024
0030-6665/24/© 2024 Elsevier Inc. All rights reserved.

oto.theclinics.com

studies are limited to specific conditions and case reports. In addition, patients with dysphagia will often have multiple comorbidities and therefore it is challenging to isolate the impact of metabolic disorders on dysphagia.

Thyroid Disorders

Thyroid disorders are common endocrine disorders that can occasionally cause dysphagia. Thyroid hormone disorders both hyper and hypo can result in myopathy. The pathogenesis of myopathy in thyroid dysfunction is not well understood, however, it is due to a result of processes affecting muscle function and metabolism. Thyroid dysfunction can cause skeletal muscle weakness and reduced and slowed muscle contraction which can result in dysphagia. Thyroid dysfunction can result in enlargement of the thyroid gland; this can create external compression of the hypopharynx and esophagus which results in dysphagia.

Hyperthyroidism

Hyperthyroidism will typically present as a constellation of symptoms including weight loss, tachycardia, tremors, heat intolerance, and diarrhea. Hyperthyroidism as a cause of dysphagia (or at least isolated dysphagia) is rare.

Hyperthyroidism can result in myopathy of pharyngeal and esophageal muscles, as well as electrolyte disturbances affecting the skeletal muscles. Myopathy due to thyroxine excess is thought to be due to an increase muscle metabolism and breakdown at a rate that is faster than it can be replaced. The more severe the excess (such as in thyroid storm), the more pronounced the muscle breakdown and myopathy. Electrolytes can also be deranged in thyrotoxicosis that could exacerbate myopathy. Evaluation with video fluoroscopic swallow study and esophagram will often show oropharyngeal and esophageal dysfunction. Aspiration can also frequently be identified, and examination of a cohort of 20 patients with dysphagia and thyrotoxicosis >30% had an associated episode of aspiration pneumonia.[1] Classically, patients with dysphagia in the setting of hyperthyroidism were improved substantially with the return of a euthyroid state.[1–3]

Hypothyroidism

Hypothyroidism is most commonly the result of Hashimoto's thyroiditis, an autoimmune condition resulting in chronic lymphocytic infiltration of the thyroid gland. Patients with hypothyroidism will often have weight gain, hair thinning, fatigue, cold intolerance, constipation, and skin changes. Dysphagia can occur because of multiple processes with hypothyroidism. It can cause myopathy of the muscles involved with swallowing, alterations in esophageal motility, neurogenic discoordination of swallowing muscles as well as physical infiltration of these muscles with myxedema.

Hypothyroidism can cause myopathies causing muscle cramps, weakness, and generalized aches, affecting not only proximal skeletal muscles, but also muscles involved with swallowing. Patients will frequently suffer with slowed gastric motility, delayed gastric emptying, dyspepsia, and gastroesophageal reflux disease as a result of hormonal effects on motility.[4] Oropharyngeal dysfunction due to neurogenic dysphagia can also result. Video fluoroscopy will show disorganized swallow and often associated with aspiration.[5] Manometry may reveal a reduced amplitude and duration of peristalsis. Much like hyperthyroidism, return to a euthyroid state will frequently treat dysphagia and esophageal symptoms of hypothyroidism.[6]

Case reports have revealed a rare manifestation of hypothyroidism, with myxedematous infiltration of the cricopharyngeus leading to oropharyngeal dysphagia. Video fluoroscopic and manometric studies highlight a fixed, high-amplitude pressure at the level of the cricopharyngeus that returned to normal after thyroid replacement therapy.[7,8]

Physical compression associated with a thyroid goiter can occur because of either hypo or hyperthyroidism. Compression by a goiter causing dysphagia and airway symptoms is an indication for surgical resection with total thyroidectomy. Congenital lingual thyroids have also presented as primary dysphagia.[9]

Diagnostic tests and work-up. To evaluate thyroid dysfunction, a thyroid panel can be ordered including thyroid-stimulating hormone and free T thyroxine (T4), thyroid peroxidase antibodies (TPO antibodies), and thyroglobulin antibodies (TG antibodies). These provide information on thyroid function, amount of circulating hormone, and high antibodies which can be elevated in auto-immune thyroid disorders (Graves and Hashimotos). Thyroglobulin is more useful in monitoring in thyroid carcinoma, but is usually part of the panel. Thyroid-binding globulin is a measure of thyroid hormone transport, and can be abnormal in some rare genetic conditions, liver failure, and high estrogen/testosterone levels. Free T3 can be ordered; it is the more biologically active form of thyroid hormone, but a much smaller proportion of the circulating hormone. It provides information about metabolism. In addition to the thyroid panel, you could consider a thyroid ultrasound. Referral to endocrinology is then recommended.

Parathyroid Disorders

Parathyroid disorders can contribute to dysphagia through its effects on calcium levels and the subsequent neuromuscular excitability. Calcium homeostasis is tightly regulated by parathyroid hormone and vitamin D. The balance of these hormones will either promote calcium resorption or excretion in the kidney and small intestine, and either bone resorption or osteoclastic release.

Hyperparathyroidism

Hyperparathyroidism can be primary as in instances of parathyroid hormone (PTH) secreting adenoma, or secondary in the setting of parathyroid gland hyperplasia resulting from vitamin D deficiency, chronic kidney disease, and hypocalcemia. Hypercalcemia can cause myopathies with muscle weakness and hyporeflexia that can result in dysphagia. Calcium effects on swallowing muscle function are summarized in **Table 1** below. Parathyroid adenomas, the most common cause of hyperparathyroidism, are benign growths of 1 or more of the parathyroid glands. They are typically small (average size of ~2 cm) and weigh roughly 1 g; however, there have been a number of reports of very large adenomas presenting primarily as dysphagia.[10–13]

Hypoparathyroidism

Hypoparathyroidism is more rare and can be seen in iatrogenic states (post thyroidectomy or parathyroidectomy), congenital (chromosome 22q11 microdeletion syndrome), and in autoimmune conditions such as part of autoimmune polyendocrine syndromes. Hypocalcemia can result and frequently presents with muscle twitching and paresthesias; however, can progress to develop tetany if severe and untreated. Dysphagia has been reported with hypocalcemia, possibly due to inappropriate muscle contractility and coordination.[14,15]

Diagnostic tests and work-up. If you suspect a parathyroid disorder based on history and examination, the next step is to order several diagnostic laboratory tests, including serum calcium, serum intact parathyroid hormone, renal function tests, and phosphorous and vitamin D levels. These will often guide you to a likely diagnosis. A neck ultrasound can be used to identify water-clear cell hyperplasia, 4 gland hypertrophy in renal

Table 1
Electrolyte imbalances and their impact on swallowing function

Electrolyte	High	Low
Calcium	Hypercalcemia increases nerve depolarization threshold leading to muscle weakness. • Dysphagia secondary to muscle weakness has been reported, and is typically reversed with normalization of calcium.[42,43]	Hypocalcemia can cause neuromuscular irritability, muscle spasm, and in severe instances, tetany. • Dysphagia can result from myopathy in the setting of hypocalcemia.[14]
Magnesium	Does not usually cause true dysphagia.	Low magnesium levels are associated with neuromuscular excitability and muscle weakness. The following can result. • Pharyngeal and hypopharyngeal muscle dysfunction.[44] • Reduced esophageal peristalsis.[45] • Diffuse esophageal spasm.[46] All of these can be identified on modified barium swallow study or esophagram and are typically reversed with the use of intramuscular magnesium.
Potassium	Dysphagia is not well described	Dysphagia is not well described
Sodium	Does not usually cause true dysphagia.	Hyponatremia itself does not typically cause dysphagia. However, inappropriate rapid correction can cause severe dysphagia, amongst a myriad of other severe symptoms. • Rapid correction of hyponatremia can lead to central pontine myelinolysis , causing pseudo bulbar palsy with severe dysphagia, dysarthria, quadriplegia

failure, and also can identify parathyroid adenoma. If concern for parathyroid adenoma and no findings on ultrasound, you can also consider ordering a sestamibi scan (parathyroid scintigraphy) which uses a radioactive tracer to localize abnormally metabolic parathyroid glands. A dual-energy X-ray absorptiometry bone density scan is also important due to risk of osteoporosis with hyperparathyroidism.

Diabetes Mellitus

Diabetes is a chronic endocrine disorder characterized by hyperglycemia and either the inability to produce insulin or insulin resistance. It frequently results in macrovascular and microvascular disease, manifesting as peripheral, cardiovascular, and cerebrovascular disease and downstream neuropathy, nephropathy, and retinopathy.[16]

Dysphagia in the diabetic population is a relatively common complaint, with over a quarter of patients suffering from difficulty swallowing.[17] The neuropathy seen in diabetes can result in esophageal dysmotility, gastroparesis, and increased presence of gastroesophageal reflux.[18] Patients with diabetes may also be more prone to oropharyngeal dysphagia, although this is less well established.[19] Dysphagia in this population classically presents as solid food dysphagia, slow swallow, chest discomfort with swallowing, acid taste and/or heart burn, nausea, vomiting, bloating, and early satiation.[20]

Esophageal dysmotility in diabetes mellitus

Diabetes mellitus both type 1 and type 2 are associated with microvascular disease and neuropathy as complication of this disease process. Neuropathy affects not only the peripheral sensory nerves but also affects the motor and autonomic nerves.[21,22] There is an estimated prevalence of neuropathy in roughly 15% to 25% of patients with diabetes mellitus.[23,24] Esophageal dysmotility in patients with diabetes appears to be a result of a combination of diabetic autonomic neuropathy (DAN) and diabetic motor neuropathy.[18]

DAN has been shown to result in vagal nerve dysfunction, which is thought to be the primary cause of esophageal dysmotility issues in patients with diabetes.[21] High-resolution manometry will frequently detect reduced lower esophageal sphincter (LES) pressure, reduced amplitude contractions, reduced number of peristaltic waves, reduced speed of peristalsis, impaired esophageal transit, and poorly coordinated or spastic contractions. Patients can also have impaired relaxation during swallowing and asynchronous or repetitive contractions.[25] Patients with more diabetic complications had a higher incidence of esophageal motility disorders.[26] This process contributes to abnormal gastroesophageal reflux secondary to lower LES pressure and increased transient relaxations of the LES. The prevalence of gastric reflux is much higher in patients with diabetes compared to the general population, with close to 30% of patients with diabetes having reflux on 24 hour ambulatory pH probe testing.[27]

Lifestyle modification is a cornerstone in the management of diabetic esophageal pathology. Reducing intake of high-glycemic index foods can be helpful to reduce transient hyperglycemia and its effect on the LES. Small, soft, and more frequent meals can be helpful in managing the symptoms of esophageal dysmotility. Avoidance of triggering foods, timing of eating, and sleeping position can be helpful in symptomatic reflux disease. There are numerous medications that are used in the management of diabetes including metformin, sodium-glucose cotransporter 2 inhibitors (eg, empagliflozin or Jardiance$_{TM}$), and glucagon-like peptide-1 (GLP-1) agonists (eg, semaglutide or Ozempic$_{TM}$) which are all considered first line. GLP-1 medications act to stimulate insulin release, inhibit glucagon release, and suppress appetite by slowing of gastric emptying and affecting central neural mechanisms of appetite. The use of GLP-1 medications has sky-rocketed in the last few years.[28] Of note, their consumption causes gastroparesis, nausea and reflux, and these in turn can increase dysphagia. These consequences can be quite profound; anecdotally these have resulted in increasing incidence of regurgitation and reflux during anesthetic induction, which has led to new anesthesia guidelines recommending holding this medication between 1 and 7 days prior to a general anesthetic.[29]

Diagnostic tests and work-up. Fore patients who do not yet have a diagnosis but you suspect diabetes, there are a number of investigations you can order. A fasting glucose of 126 mg/dL or higher indicates the presence of diabetes, and 100 to 125 mg/dL reflects a pre-diabetic state. Random glucose is less effective in diagnosing diabetes, however, a result of >200 mg/mL is concerning for diabetes. Glycated hemoglobin (HbA1)c is glycated form of hemoglobin and offers an estimate of blood glucose levels over the prior 3 months. A HbA1c of >6.5% (48 mmol/mol) is concerning for diabetes, 5.7% to 6.4% (39–46 mmol/mol) reflects a pre-diabetic state. Urinary glucose and ketones is no longer used in diagnosis due to being an indirect measure, not specific, and the threshold for detection is high (blood levels need to be 180 to 200 mg/dL in order to detect). Screening for kidney function with creatinine and blood urea nitrogen (BUN) could be considered as a measure of end-organ dysfunction. Once identified, a referral to endocrinology and input from a diabetes educator or nurse is recommended.

Cushing Disease and Syndrome

Cushing disease (CD) is the result of excessive secretion of adrenocorticotrophic hormone (ACTH) by a pituitary adenoma. This stimulates the adrenal gland to produce excess amounts of cortisol. Cushing syndrome (CS) is the constellation of "cushingoid" symptoms that arise from excessive glucocorticoids, which can be caused by CD, as well as exogenous glucocorticoids. These symptoms include truncal obesity, proximal muscle weakness, lipodystrophy, skin striae, and osteoporosis. Whilst dysphagia is not commonly cited as a side effect of Cushing disease or syndrome, there have been reports of dysphagia as a presenting complaint.[30] The hypothesized underlying reason is myopathy and connective tissue changes that occur with CS. In addition, there is an association between CD and hypothyroidism due to pituitary hypofunction, which can also promote dysphagia.

Diagnostic tests and work-up

A careful assessment of the patient's medical history and medication history may point to Cushing syndrome. If concerned for Cushing syndrome, you can order a 24-hour urinary free cortisol and or a midnight salivary cortisol test. A high-dose dexamethasone suppression test can be used to distinguish Cushing syndrome from Cushing disease (Cushing syndrome does not get suppressed by high- dose dexamethasone). If concerned about Cushing disease, you could also order plasma ACTH and ACTH stimulation test. MRI of the brain to evaluate the pituitary and computed tomography (CT) abdomen to evaluate for adrenal gland tumors can be done. If any of these assessments are abnormal, it would be prudent to refer to endocrinology.

Diffuse Idiopathic Skeletal Hyperostosis

Diffuse idiopathic skeletal hyperostosis (DISH), also known as Forestier's Syndrome, is a systemic condition that causes osseous changes at the connective tissue insertion of tendons and ligaments to bone. DISH is considered a rheumatologic disorder; however, there is a hypothesized shared inflammatory pathway involving metabolic syndrome.[31] Metabolic disturbances appear to be highly associated with the development of DISH, with metabolic syndrome, obesity, and visceral adipose tissue being strong risk factors for the development of DISH, and as such DISH has been included amongst this chapter as a cause metabolic cause for dysphagia.

The condition is more common in males and has a higher incidence in western populations.[32] New bone formation and remodeling at these entheseal sites are governed by changes in fibroblasts, chondrocytes, collagen, and matrix, and are affected by circulating numbers of specific cytokines and adipokines.[33] DISH is characterized by boney bridges on the anterolateral spine, most commonly the thoracic and cervical spine. Whilst many patients are asymptomatic, dysphagia is a common presentation of DISH.

Dysphagia in DISH is primarily a result of altered physical mechanics, with protruding osteophytes impacting the swallowing mechanism. Classically, patients will report solid food dysphagia that gradually worsens; they may also report foreign body or globus sensation. The protrusion of these osseous lesions at the level of the cervical spine can impinge the mobility of the pharynx and epiglottis and prevent a food bolus from easily entering the post cricoid space and the upper esophagus. **Fig. 1** reveals characteristic distal chip flexible laryngoscopy and modified barium swallow study appearance.

Pre-operative appearance of flexible laryngoscopy and modified barium swallow study (MBSS) in a patient with Diffuse Idiopathic Skeletal Hyperostosis (DISH)

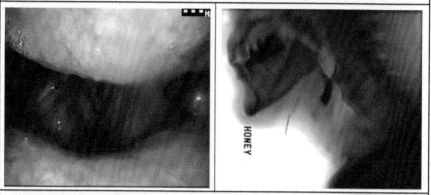

Post-operative appearance of the same patient's flexible laryngoscopy and modified barium swallow study (MBSS)

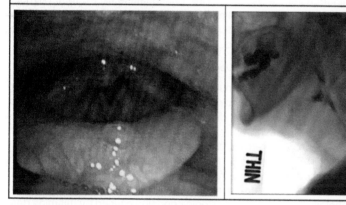

Fig. 1. Flexible laryngoscopy and modified barium swallow study assessment in diffuse idiopathic skeletal hyperostosis (DISH). Characteristic appearance pre-surgical and post-surgical excision of cervical osteophytes in DISH. The first set of images show cervical osteophytes protruding and premature contact of epiglottis with posterior pharynx with food bolus remaining in the vallecula. After surgical excision, there is no longer visible fullness on laryngoscopy and now improved passage of the food bolus.

If dysphagia is severe, enough treatment is with an anterior approach to the cervical spine and osteophytectomy. In milder cases, swallow therapy, diet modification, and anti-inflammatory therapies can be used.[34] Surgical excision is the only treatment that will provide curative management of the dysphagia; however, the approach to the cervical spine will likely worsen swallowing in the acute period, and may potentially have long-term laryngeal or pharyngeal dysfunction.[35] By 3 months post operatively, most patients report significant improvements in swallowing compared to preoperative function.

Diagnostic tests and work-up
Evaluating for DISH from an otolaryngology perspective will be based initially on clinical suspicion on flexible laryngoscopy with the presence of firm prominences at the

posterior pharynx and hypopharynx near the esophageal inlet. The next step in evaluation is a modified barium swallow study to look at the cervical spine and how this relates to the mechanics of swallowing. If there are multiple sites of calcification within the anterior longitudinal ligament of the cervical spine, it is reasonable to suspect DISH. Due to the relationship between DISH and metabolic syndrome, a screening evaluation with HbA1c, fasting glucose, lipid profile, and renal function tests and a referral to primary care physician or internal medicine is recommended.

Electrolyte Disturbances

Dysphagia leading to dehydration, inadequate oral intake, and in severe cases, malnutrition is a frequent cause of electrolyte derangement. Less commonly derangements in electrolyte levels can result in symptomatic dysphagia. **Table 1** below provides a summary of the effects of different electrolyte imbalances on swallowing function.

Diagnostic tests and work-up
If concerned for electrolyte dysfunction, then you should consider ordering a complete metabolic panel (CMP) which includes sodium (Na), potassium (K), chloride (Cl), glucose, creatinine, BUN, liver function tests including alanine aminotransferase (ALT), aspartate aminotransferase (AST), alkaline phosphatase (ALP), total bilirubin, and albumin. Serum calcium, ionized calcium, magnesium, and phosphate levels are not part of the CMP and should be done separately. Depending on the results, involving internal medicine early is advised.

Wernicke's Encephalopathy and Alcohol Dependence

Heavy alcohol consumption can lead to numerous severe health problems, ranging from organ dysfunction in the form of liver cirrhosis, cardiomyopathy, and pancreatitis, and significant neurologic and cognitive disorders including dementia, Wernicke's encephalopathy, and Korsakoff syndrome. Alcohol dependence is associated with periods of acute intoxication, long-term tolerance to alcohol, and symptoms of physical dependence. Chronic malnutrition is also commonly seen as part of alcohol dependence, with reduced caloric intake, poorer absorption of nutrients and increased protein catabolism and reduced synthesis.

Wernicke's encephalopathy (WE) is a neurologic condition caused by thiamine deficiency and presents with a typical triad of ataxia, confusion, and ophthalmoplegia. Alcohol dependence or even just severe malnutrition can result in thiamine deficiency and characteristic lesions in the thalamus, hypothalamus, mammillary bodies, and midbrain. Dysphagia is a rare symptom of WE; however, a systematic review found 13 case reports of patients with WE and dysphagia, and revealed that dysphagia was a primary presenting symptom in 9 (69.3%).[36] Dysphagia seems to be oropharyngeal in origin, with patients reporting difficulty with initiation of swallow.[37] The pathogenesis of dysphagia is unclear; 1 hypothesis is that it is be due to dysfunction of the cranial nerves located in the floor of the fourth ventricle, namely IX, X, and XII.[36,37] Treatment along with supportive care is thiamine replacement, and will typically result in significant improvement in swallowing within a few days of administration.

Diagnostic tests and work-up
Evaluation of WE should be performed in the inpatient hospital setting, as this is considered a medical emergency. If you are seeing a patient in your clinic with the afore-mentioned symptoms and you suspect WE, you could order thiamine levels and a CMP and concurrently organize for hospital admission and further work up. MRI of the brain may reveal the characteristic changes including thalamic, mammillary body, and periaqueductal hyperintense signals reflecting edema and gliosis. Critical

care, internal medicine, and psychiatry should all play a role in the care of patients with WE.

Malnutrition

Malnutrition is a common sequela of dysphagia; however, the metabolic processes that result from malnutrition also encourage dysphagia independently.

Dysphagia and frailty

Dysphagia in the elderly as a result of frailty and malnutrition has been termed "sarcopenic dysphagia."[38] This is characterized by oropharyngeal and laryngeal muscle atrophy and weakness associated with overall physical deconditioning and functional decline. This can encourage a cycle where these patients avoid challenging foods or anything requiring mastication resulting in further nutritional deficiency, atrophy, and decline.[38] This process is often catalyzed by a hospital admission.

Critical illness

For all patients (not just elderly), critical illness and hospital admission is associated with significant muscle atrophy, including of the oropharynx and larynx. Systematic reviews estimate that critically ill patients will lose 2% of their muscle mass per day in the first week of being in an intensive care unit (ICU).[39,40] In addition to this, especially in an ICU setting, patients with swallowing difficulties will be placed on a tube-fed diet or parenteral nutrition, and not permitted an oral diet further exacerbating muscle atrophy, loss of strength, and coordination.

In both patient populations described, there is frequently clinically evident muscle wasting in the base of tongue, pharynx, and larynx. Patients will also develop bowing of the vocal folds and an elliptical-shaped glottic gap reflecting atrophy. This combined with reduced functional capacity and cough strength increases the risk of aspiration. For these patients, the authors recommend intentional oral care, nutritional supplements, intensive physical and swallowing therapy, and as long as safe maintaining an oral diet as much as possible.[40] In the setting of a glottic gap and evidence of aspiration, a bilateral vocal fold augmentation with temporary filler injection can also be helpful.[41]

Diagnostic tests and work-up

There are a number of laboratory tests that should be ordered if you suspect malnutrition including complete blood count (CBC) which reveals anemia, common in malnutrition. Serum albumin and pre-albumin reflect nutritional status, with pre-albumin being more sensitive to changes in acute malnutrition. Total protein and complete metabolic panel reveals electrolyte levels and liver and renal function. Thyroid function tests can be abnormal as malnutrition can affect thyroid hormone production. Serum calcium, ionized calcium, magnesium, phosphate, vitamin levels (vitamin D, B12, folate, zinc, and iron) should be ordered and are often abnormal in malnutrition. C-reactive protein (CRP) can be elevated in malnutrition, especially if underlying inflammatory or infectious disorders. Evaluation by internal medicine and dietician is needed.

SUMMARY

Swallowing is a complex neuromuscular process with precise coordination required for successful swallow. Disruptions in any of these processes can cause significant dysphagia, making dysphagia a common manifestation of systemic diseases. These disorders can lead to muscular weakness, muscle spasm, muscle atrophy, and motility disorders, all with effects on the swallowing mechanism. Treatment of the underlying illness and hormonal or electrolyte derangement usually results in return of normal or baseline swallow.

CLINICS CARE POINTS

- Dysphagia is a common manifestation of endocrine and metabolic disorders.
- Typically, the cause of the dysphagia is a result of processes affecting muscular strength and coordination, including neuropathy, myopathy, and dysmotility.
- Evaluation is guided by underlying condition and nature of the patient symptoms; however, use of 1 or more studies including modified barium swallow study, esophagram, high-resolution manometry, and pH and impedance probe testing is usually recommended.
- Management of dysphagia is usually routed in tight control of the underlying cause and normalization of homeostasis.
- There is a role for swallow therapy (especially in deconditioned, critically ill, and malnourished patients) and optimization of associated symptoms (eg, acid reflux)

DISCLOSURE

The authors have no relevant disclosures.

REFERENCES

1. Alwithenani R, Andrade DM, Zhang L, et al. Myopathic dysphagia caused by thyrotoxicosis: a case report and review of the literature. Endocrinol Diabetes Metab Case Rep 2022. ID21–0175.
2. Chiu WY, Yang CC, Huang IC, et al. Dysphagia as a manifestation of thyrotoxicosis: report of three cases and literature review. Dysphagia 2004;19:120–4.
3. Greenblatt DY, Sippel R, Leverson G, et al. Thyroid resection improves perception of swallowing function in patients with thyroid disease. World J Surg 2009; 33(2):255–60.
4. Kahraman H, Kaya N, Demirçali A, et al. Gastric emptying time in patients with primary hypothyroidism. Eur J Gastroenterol Hepatol 1997;9(9):901–4.
5. Urquhart AD, Rea IM, Lawson LT, et al. A new complication of hypothyroid coma: neurogenic dysphagia: presentation, diagnosis, and treatment. Thyroid 2001; 11(6):595–8.
6. Ebert EC. The thyroid and the gut. J Clin Gastroenterol 2010;44(6):402–6.
7. Wright RA, Penner DB. Myxedema and upper esophageal dysmotility. Dig Dis Sci 1981;26(4):376–7.
8. Reiss M. Dysphagia as a symptom of myxedema. Praxis 1998;87(18):627–9.
9. Toso A, Colombani F, Averono G, et al. Lingual thyroid causing dysphagia and dyspnoea. Case reports and review of the literature. Acta Otorhinolaryngol Ital 2009;29(4):213–7.
10. Ulanovski D, Feinmesser R, Cohen M, et al. Preoperative evaluation of patients with parathyroid adenoma: role of high-resolution ultrasonography. Head Neck 2002;24(1):1–5.
11. Ahsayen FZ, Haddadi Z, Aggari HE, et al. Dysphagia revealing a giant cystic parathyroid adenoma. Radiol Case Rep 2022;17(10):3556–8.
12. Muelleman T, Yalamanchali S, Shnayder Y. Bilateral pyriform sinus parathyroid adenomas. Ear Nose Throat J 2018;97(3):E38–40.

13. Ziaeean B, Sohrabi-Nazari S. Huge parathyroid adenoma with dysphagia presentation; a case report from southern iran. Iran J Med Sci 2016;41(5):446–9.

14. Thomas C, Bhamra N, Darr A, et al. Simultaneous dysphagia and stridor: an unreported presentation of hypocalcaemia. J Surg Case Rep 2020;2020(9):317.

15. Ratanaanekchai T, Art-smart T, Vatanasapt P. Dysphagia after total laryngectomy resulting from hypocalcemia: case report. J Med Assoc Thai 2004;87(6):722–4.

16. Papatheodorou K, Banach M, Bekiari E, et al. Complications of diabetes 2017. J Diabetes Res 2018;1–4. Article ID 3086167.

17. Feldman M, Schiller LR. Disorders of gastrointestinal motility associated with diabetes mellitus. Ann Intern Med 1983;98(3):378–84.

18. Kinekawa F, Kubo F, Matsuda K, et al. Relationship between esophageal dysfunction and neuropathy in diabetic patients. Am J Gastroenterol 2001;96(7):2026–32.

19. Zakaria DA, Bekhet MM, Khodeir MS, et al. Oropharyngeal dysphagia and diabetes mellitus: screening of 200 type 1 and type 2 patients in Cairo, Egypt. Folia Phoniatr Logop 2018;70:134–7.

20. Boltin D, Zvidi I, Steinmetz A, et al. Vomiting and dysphagia predict delayed gastric emptying in diabetic and nondiabetic subjects. J Diabetes Res 2014;1–7. Article ID 294032.

21. Watkins PJ. Diabetic autonomic neuropathy. N Engl J Med 1990;322:1078–9.

22. Abrahamsson H. Gastrointestinal motility disorders in patients with diabetes mellitus. J Int Med 1995;237:403–9.

23. Abbott CA, Malik RA, van Ross ER, et al. Prevalence and characteristics of painful diabetic neuropathy in a large community-based diabetic population in the UK. Diabetes Care 2011;34(10):2220–4.

24. Davies M, Brophy S, Williams R, et al. The prevalence, severity, and impact of painful diabetic peripheral neuropathy in type 2 diabetes. Diabetes Care 2006; 29(7):1518–22.

25. Portincasa P, Bonfrate L, Wang DQH, et al. Novel insights into the pathogenic impact of diabetes on the gastrointestinal tract. Eur J Clin Invest 2022;52:e13846.

26. Muroi K, Miyaahara R, Funasaka K, et al. Comparison of high-resolution manometry in patients complaining of dysphagia among patients with or without diabetes mellitus. Digestion 2021;102:554–62.

27. Lluch I, Ascaso JF, Mora F, et al. Gastroesophageal reflux in diabetes mellitus. Am J Gastroenterol 1999;94:919–24.

28. Adhikari R, Jha K, Dardari Z, et al. National trends in use of sodium-glucose cotransporter-2 inhibitors and glucagon-like peptide-1 receptor agonists by cardiologists and other specialties, 2015 to 2020. J Am Heart Assoc 2022;11(9):e023811.

29. Joshi GP, Abdelmalak BB, Weigel WA, et al. American Society of Anesthesiologists Practice Guidelines for Preoperative Fasting: Carbohydrate-containing Clear Liquids with or without Protein, Chewing Gum, and Pediatric Fasting Duration-A Modular Update of the 2017 American Society of Anesthesiologists Practice Guidelines for Preoperative Fasting. Anesthesiology 2023;138(2):132–51.

30. Kuan EC, Peng KA, Suh JD, et al. Otolaryngic manifestations of Cushing disease. Ear Nose Throat J 2017;96(8):E28–30.

31. Harlianto NI, Westerink J, Foppen W, et al. Visceral adipose tissue and different measures of adiposity in different severities of diffuse idiopathic skeletal hyperostosis. J Personalized Med 2021;11(7):663–75.

32. Mesolella M, Buono S, D'Aniello R, et al. Diffuse idiopathic skeletal hyperostosis (dish): role of logopedic rehabilitation in dysphagia. J Personalized Med 2023; 13(6):994–1106.

33. Kuperus JS, Mohamed Hoesein FAA, de Jong PA, et al. Diffuse idiopathic skeletal hyperostosis: Etiology and clinical relevance. Best Pract Res Clin Rheumatol 2020;34(3):101527–40.

34. Ohki M. Dysphagia due to Diffuse Idiopathic Skeletal Hyperostosis. Case Rep Otolaryngol 2012;2012:123825.

35. Scholz C, Naseri Y, Hohenhaus M, et al. Long-term results after surgical treatment of diffuse idiopathic skeletal hyperostosis (DISH) causing dysphagia. J Clin Neurosci 2019;67:151–5.

36. Cornea A, Lata I, Simu M, et al. Wernicke encephalopathy presenting with dysphagia: a case report and systematic literature review. Nutrients 2022;14(24):5294.

37. Truedsson M, Ohlsson B, Sjöberg K. Wernicke's encephalopathy presenting with severe dysphagia: a case report. Alcohol Alcohol 2002;37(3):295–6.

38. de Sire A, Ferrillo M, Lippi L, et al. Sarcopenic dysphagia, malnutrition, and oral frailty in elderly: a comprehensive review. Nutrients 2022;14(5):982.

39. Koukourikos K, Tswaloglidou A, Kourkouta L. Muscle atrophy in intensive care unit patients. Acta Inform Med 2014;22(6):406–10.

40. Fazzini B, Markl T, Costas C, et al. The rate and assessment of muscle wasting during critical illness: a systematic review and meta-analysis. Crit Care 2023;27(1):2.

41. Giraldez-Rodriguez LA, Johns MM 3rd. Glottal insufficiency with aspiration risk in dysphagia. Otolaryngol Clin North Am 2013;46(6):1113–21.

42. Balcombe N. Dysphagia and hypercalcaemia. Postgrad Med J 1999;75(884):373–4.

43. Ayyathurai R, Webb DB, Rowland S, et al. Humoral hypercalcemia of penile carcinoma. Urology 2007;69(1):184, e9-e10.

44. Hamed IA, Lindeman RD. Dysphagia and vertical nystagmus in magnesium deficiency. Ann Intern Med 1978;89(2):222–3.

45. Flink EB. Dysphagia in magnesium deficiency. Ann Intern Med 1978;89(2):282.

46. Iannello S, Spina M, Leotta P, et al. Hypomagnesemia and smooth muscle contractility: diffuse esophageal spasm in an old female patient. Miner Electrolyte Metab 1998;24(5):348–56.

Inflammatory Causes of Dysphagia in Children

Marisa A. Ryan, MD, MPH[a],*, Anna Ermarth, MD, MS[b]

KEYWORDS

- Pediatric dysphagia • Inflammatory • Auto-immune
- Gastroesophageal reflux disease (GERD) • Eosinophilic esophagitis (EoE)
- Inflammatory bowel disease (IBD) • Idiopathic inflammatory myopathy

KEY POINTS

- Inflammatory causes of dysphagia in children can affect all phases of swallowing—oral, oropharyngeal, and esophageal.
- Most inflammatory causes of dysphagia in children are chronic and require ongoing management.
- The presence of dysphagia can portend a more severe presentation or worse prognosis for an underlying autoimmune inflammatory condition.
- Consultations with gastroenterology, allergy/immunology, rheumatology, licensed therapists, and dietetics are indicated when a chronic inflammatory cause of dysphagia is suspected.

INTRODUCTION

Inflammatory causes of dysphagia in children are varied and can include atopic, immunologic, caustic injury, and post-viral effects (**Box 1**). Since many of the underlying causes of inflammatory dysphagia in children are rare and expression of dysphagia is often given by a caregiver's observation, there is limited published epidemiology on symptomatic inflammatory causes in children. However, the epidemiology of some known inflammatory conditions and diseases that may cause dysphagia is better studied. Typically, inflammatory causes of dysphagia lead to oral phase, pharyngeal phase, or esophageal phase swallowing deficits, and many children can be affected by impairments with more than 1 or all phases of swallowing. The diagnostic workup and management recommendations vary and are often multidisciplinary. Most of

[a] Pediatric Otolaryngology, Peak ENT Associates, 1055 North 300 West, Suite 401, Provo, UT 84604, USA; [b] Department of Pediatrics, Division of Pediatric Gastroenterology, Hepatology and Nutrition, University of Utah School of Medicine, 81 Mario Capecchi Drive, Salt Lake City, UT 84113, USA
* Corresponding author.
E-mail address: Marisa.a.ryan@gmail.com

Otolaryngol Clin N Am 57 (2024) 669–684
https://doi.org/10.1016/j.otc.2024.03.002
oto.theclinics.com

Box 1
Inflammatory causes of dysphagia in children

Gastroesophageal reflux disease (GERD)

Laryngopharyngeal reflux (LPR)

Eosinophilic esophagitis (EoE)

Lymphocytic esophagitis (LE)

Irritable bowel disease (IBD)
    Ulcerative colitis (UC)
    Crohn's disease (CD)

Juvenile scleroderma
    Juvenile systemic sclerosis (jSSc)
    Juvenile localized scleroderma (jLS)

Sjögren's syndrome (SS)

Idiopathic inflammatory myopathies
    Juvenile dermatomyositis (JDM)
    Juvenile polymyositis (JPM)

Infectious mucositis

Multi-system inflammatory syndrome (MIS-C)/pediatric inflammatory multisystem syndrome (PIMS)

Caustic ingestion

---

the underlying conditions are chronic, require long-term management, and have varied outcomes.

GASTROESOPHAGEAL REFLUX DISEASE

Gastroesophageal reflux (GER) is a common condition especially in infants and young children with a peak in incidence at 4 months of age affecting 67% of infants and then a decline to 5% at 10 to 12 months of age.[1] In most infants and children, GER is a benign physiologic process that improves with time and patient development out of infancy. This common physiologic process differs from gastroesophageal reflux disease (GERD), which has accompanying complications and affects 2% to 7% of children.[2] In older children age 3 to 18 years, the incidence of pathologic GERD increases again and ranges from 1.8% to 25%. Overall, it is estimated that 1.8% to 8.2% of children have GERD.[3] A GERD diagnosis is usually based on history and physical, but sometimes additional testing with endoscopy, esophageal pH, and impedence testing are indicated.

The esophageal GERD complications that can affect swallowing function include esophagitis and fibrosing esophageal/peptic strictures.[3] Histologically, GER inflammation can involve both eosinophilic and neutrophilic mixed cells in surface epithelium.[3] With this mixed cell infiltration, prolonged esophagitis can also lead to esophageal dysmotility.[3]

First-line treatment includes dietary/feeding modifications such as smaller meal volumes or trials of extensively hydrolyzed formula in babies, positioning modifications, thickening of feeds, and lifestyle modifications where possible.[3] Medical management with histamine-2 receptor antagonists, proton pump inhibitors (PPIs), or topical antacids, and anti-reflux fundoplication surgeries should all be reserved for intractable GERD with risk of chronic esophagitis.[3,4] When this occurs, most severe of cases

GERD can lead to esophageal stricture or narrowing and requires balloon or bougie dilation,[5,6] esophageal stenting,[6,7] or sleeve stricture resection.[5] It can rarely lead to esophageal obliteration requiring a rendezvous procedure to re-cannulate[8] or an esophageal replacement with stomach or intestinal conduits.[5] Fundoplication should be reserved for the most severe cases or for neurologically-impaired children, as, unfortunately, fundoplication procedures can lead to additional dysphagia due to obstruction of the distal esophagus as a child ages and cannot be reversed.[1,9] Alternatives to fundoplication can include transpyloric feeding and this is a viable option for chronic GERD management with similar long-term outcomes.[10]

LARYNGOPHARYNGEAL REFLUX

Reflux contents can also extend above the upper esophageal sphincter to the pharyngeal and laryngeal tissues in a distinct condition called "laryngopharyngeal reflux (LPR)."[11] In general, young children tend to have relatively more extension of refluxate up into the pharynx compared to adults as seen by more frequent regurgitation.[12] Traditional heartburn and GER symptoms are often absent in LPR. LPR can present with laryngitis[13] and can reduce laryngeal mucosal sensation leading to inflammatory, oropharyngeal dysphagia.[14,15] These sensory deficits can improve with treatment of the reflux with medical or surgical management[14,16] and the associated dysphagia may also improve.[16]

Oropharyngeal dysphagia including aspiration and reflux are strongly associated with laryngomalacia.[1,2,17] Laryngomalacia is the most common congenital laryngeal aberration in children and is due to supraglottic structure collapse. There is an association between laryngomalacia and increased supraglottic pepsin from laryngopharyngeal reflux[18] as well as supraglottic inflammatory mucosal changes suggesting GER,[19] but it is not entirely clear if GER is causative. A systematic review of 6 studies with meta-analysis of 5 of them by Rossoni and colleagues showed high study heterogeneity, but a 59% reduction in oropharyngeal dysphagia after supraglottoplasty for laryngomalacia.[17] However, patients with laryngomalacia can still have dysphagia postoperatively and some studies even indicate a higher risk of dysphagia and hospitalization after supraglottoplasty.[20–22] Reflux symptoms often improve after supraglottoplasty; however, it is less clear if outcomes improve due to surgery, additional thickening of feeds, or concomitant anti-reflux medications in infants with laryngomalacia.[23,24] Thickened feeds has been shown to have a protective effect against further hospitalization for respiratory causes post-supraglottoplasty, while patients on anti-reflux medications showed worse post-procedure outcomes.[22]

EOSINOPHILIC ESOPHAGITIS

Since the first report in 1978 by Landres and colleagues,[25] eosinophilic esophagitis (EoE) has become an increasingly more recognized cause of esophagitis and dysphagia. It is present world-wide but has been studied most in western countries. It most commonly affects Caucasian, non-Hispanic men initially presenting at school-age to middle-age, but can be diagnosed as young as infancy. Per a 5-year North American population database study, pediatric incidence estimates 24 per 100,000 cases per year.[26] In a large commercial claims database, 24% of cases occurred in those less than18 year old.[27] Increased risk of EoE occurs in those with family history of atopy including atopic dermatitis, allergic rhinitis, asthma, and food allergies. While typical presenting symptoms are dysphagia to solids and esophageal food impactions, symptoms in infants and children can be nonspecific and include feeding issues, vomiting, and poor growth.

Diagnosis is made with esophagoscopy and biopsy. A validated scoring system provides a severity score based on visual findings—edema, rings, exudates, furrows, and strictures (EREFS) (**Fig. 1**).[28] A histologic criterion for diagnosis is equal to or greater than 15 eosinophils per high powered field.[29] When severe or untreated, fibrostenosis of the esophagus, intractable dysphagia symptoms, and complications of strictures or dysmotility can occur. Esophagrams can reveal narrowing and strictures and be complementary when evaluating more severe dysphagia in this population.[30]

Treatment options are listed in **Box 2**. An elemental or elimination diet can be curative in many, but for children this is often unpalatable and difficult to continue without enteral access.[31] Therefore, other successful management options have been used including swallowed corticosteroids, PPIs, and most recently the biologic dupilumab, approved for children >1 year of age. Close continuity of care and endoscopic surveillance are necessary for this chronic condition.

Atopy in other systems such as rhinosinusitis and persistent eosinophilia can be found in patients with EoE. It is challenging to determine if some of these findings are directly related to the EoE or just evidence of underlying atopy. Several studies have found that many children with EoE present first to the otolaryngologist with symptoms of chronic cough, hoarseness, globus, and airway symptoms in addition to dysphagia symptoms.[1] In a single-center study of pediatric patients seen by a multidisciplinary aerodigestive clinic, there was an association with biopsy-proven EoE with eosinophilia found on arytenoid biopsies.[32–34] The concern with chronic laryngitis, whether it be from eosinophilic inflammation, gastric reflux, or another cause is that

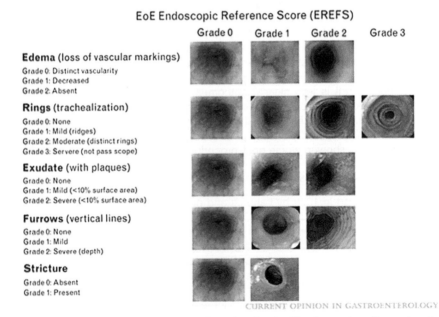

EoE Endoscopic Reference Score (EREFS)

Grade 0   Grade 1   Grade 2   Grade 3

Edema (loss of vascular markings)
Grade 0: Distinct vascularity
Grade 1: Decreased
Grade 2: Absent

Rings (trachealization)
Grade 0: None
Grade 1: Mild (ridges)
Grade 2: Moderate (distinct rings)
Grade 3: Severe (not pass scope)

Exudate (with plaques)
Grade 0: None
Grade 1: Mild (<10% surface area)
Grade 2: Severe (<10% surface area)

Furrows (vertical lines)
Grade 0: None
Grade 1: Mild
Grade 2: Severe (depth)

Stricture
Grade 0: Absent
Grade 1: Present

CURRENT OPINION IN GASTROENTEROLOGY

Fig. 1. Representative endoscopic images depicting the classification and grading system for endoscopically identified esophageal features in eosinophilic esophagitis. (*From* Kia L, Hirano I. Advances in the endoscopic evaluation of eosinophilic esophagitis. Current Opinion in Gastroenterology. 2016;32(4):325-331.)

Box 2
Treatment options for eosinophilic esophagitis

Elemental diet: amino acid-based formulas

Elimination diets
   Empiric 6-food elimination diet: avoid milk, wheat, eggs, soy, seafood, and nuts
   Empiric 4-food elimination diet: avoid milk, wheat, eggs, and soy
   Allergy testing-based elimination diet: avoid foods based on results of allergy testing

Corticosteroids: swallow budesonide or fluticasone twice a day

Proton pump inhibitors: esomeprazole, lansoprazole, omeprazole, pantoprazole, or rabeprazole twice a day

Dupilumab

Endoscopic dilation of symptomatic esophageal strictures

---

laryngeal mucosal sensation can be degraded which increases the risk of aspiration and persistent symptoms. In a small study, 9 patients had eosinophilia on arytenoid biopsies; 8 underwent modified barium swallow study (MBSS) and 2 of these demonstrated aspiration.[32] Furthermore, the average lipid-laden macrophages from concurrent bronchoalveolar lavage was elevated, which suggests possible increased aspiration in this group. Based on these findings, it is prudent to maintain a high suspicion for EoE in patients with airway and oropharyngeal dysphagia symptoms and also have a low threshold for reactive or atopic airway conditions in patients with confirmed EoE.

LYMPHOCYTIC ESOPHAGITIS

Lymphocytic esophagitis is a much less common cause of chronic esophagitis compared to EoE that was first described in 2006 by Rubio and colleagues[35] The overall incidence in children is not known. However, in a pathology study of 20 patients, 11 (55%) were 17 year old or younger[35] and it has been reported as young as age 2.[35,36] Dysphagia is the most common symptom; however, reflux, chest pain, nausea, and abdominal pain have also been reported in this condition.[37] Associations with Crohn disease, irritable bowel syndrome, celiac disease, allergies, gastritis as well as tobacco, alcohol, and drug use have been reported.[37,38] It is not yet clear if this condition is a disease entity within itself or concomitant inflammation with another disease process such as Crohn disease.[37] The association of lymphocytic esophagitis and Crohn disease appears to be stronger in children than in adult-onset disease.[38] Esophageal biopsies confirm intraepithelial lymphocytes in tissue. Treatment includes PPIs, topical steroids, and rarely, systemic steroids and esophageal dilations.[37] From the existing published report, this condition can be chronic but overall benign in nature.[37]

INFLAMMATORY BOWEL DISEASE

Patients with inflammatory bowel disease such as Crohn's disease (CD) and ulcerative colitis can present with various oral findings. One study reports 7% to 23% of pediatric patients have oral mucosal changes, dental caries, gingival and periodontal disease, xerostomia, and aphthous ulcerations.[39] These abnormalities can all contribute to oral phase dysphagia and the xerostomia may also have ensuing contributions to oropharyngeal dysphagia. CD can affect any part of the digestive tract and is more likely than ulcerative colitis to be associated with upper gastrointestinal inflammation. In children, esophageal CD is seen in 13% to 43% of patients; conversely, in adult CD, esophageal involvement occurs in only 0.2% to 11.2% of patients.[40,41] In a multi-national, multi-center analysis of esophageal CD, out of 40 patients, 18 were under age 16 year old and 47.5% of these presented with dysphagia or odynophagia.[42] Endoscopic findings can include mucosal erythema, erosions, ulcerations, strictures and rarely, an esophageal fistula. Histologic findings typically show acute and chronic inflammation as well as granulomatous changes.[42] Treatment usually consists of systemic monoclonal antibody therapy and/or topical or systemic corticosteroids. Esophageal treatment can also include PPIs and endoscopic dilation of more severe, symptomatic strictures.[42]

JUVENILE SYSTEMIC SCLEROSIS AND LOCALIZED SCLERODERMA

Juvenile scleroderma is a very rare autoimmune condition affecting 0.34 to 2.7 cases per 100,000 per year.[43] There are 2 major subtypes: juvenile systemic sclerosis and juvenile localized scleroderma. In juvenile localized scleroderma, findings are mostly limited to the skin and subdermal tissues and, in contrast, juvenile systemic sclerosis also affects internal organs.

For juvenile systemic sclerosis, there is a strong female predominance and presentation is typically in girls after age 8 years.[44] There is an association with low birthweight and being small for gestational age.[45] It is an auto-immune process that leads to progressive and chronic ischemia and then fibrosis of tissues, particularly skin and muscle. Within the esophagus, this systemic fibrosis process then leads to reduced strength or amplitude of muscular contractions and dysphagia develops.[46] Rutkowska-Sak et al. reported that 4/22 (18.2%) of patients at their center had dysphagia at disease presentation,[46] Frati-Munari et al. reported it in 3/5 (60%) of patients at their center,[47] and Misra and colleagues in 7/23 (30%) of patients at their center.[44] Dysphagia is more common in diffuse compared to localized disease and is one of the minor criteria for diagnosis of this condition.[47,48] Confirmation of symptoms is made by esophageal manometry which shows reduced caliber and amplitude of pan-esophageal contractions with both liquid and solid swallows.[49]

There is also a strong female predominance in juvenile localized scleroderma.[50] Weber and colleagues found a high incidence of reflux intra-esophageal 24-h pH probe monitoring in 9/14 (64%) with scleroderma or mixed connective tissue disease indicating an increased risk for esophagitis; however, only 3/14 (21%) reported symptoms of esophagitis or esophageal dysmotility.[51] Gauriso and colleagues evaluated 14 patients with esophageal manometry, distal esophagus 24h pH probes, and esophagoscopy and found esophageal abnormalities in 8/14 (57%) of patients.[52] This included abnormal esophageal pH findings in 7/14 (50%), esophageal dysmotility in 5/14 (36%), and esophagitis in 5/14 (36%) patients.[52] Esophageal manometry is also the gold-standard for confirmation of dysphagia symptoms.[49]

Treatment for both systemic sclerosis and localized scleroderma focuses on systemic anti-inflammatory and immunologic suppressing measures (eg, corticosteroids, intravenous immunoglobulin therapy (IVIG), monoclonal antibody therapy) to reduce inflammation in esophageal mucosal in order to restore normal motility. Dysphagia can wax and wane as an associated symptom within a patient's lifelong disease course or flares, and some severe presentations need nutritional support with a feeding tube until their condition improves and they can return to full nutrition.[43]

Tobacco use is associated with worsening gastrointestinal symptoms in scleroderma and therefore tobacco cessation or encouragement to not initiate tobacco use is important when counseling the juvenile scleroderma population with dysphagia.[53]

SJÖGREN'S SYNDROME

Sjögren's syndrome is rare in children and primarily affects females. It can be a primary syndrome or a secondary syndrome associated with other autoimmune diseases including lupus and scleroderma. The condition can contribute to oral and oropharyngeal dysphagia through xerostomia, reduced refluxed stomach acid neutralization by saliva, muscle weakness, and less frequently myositis.[54] Oral dysphagia has been reported in a young child due to xerostomia combined with the resulting dental and periodontal disease.[55] Oral lubricants and careful management by a dentist including dental rehabilitation can improve oral dysphagia.[55] Although dysphagia is not well described in the literature for pediatric patients with Sjögren's syndrome, dysphagia (in 45%–80%) as well as GERD (in 60%) are commonly reported in the adult literature.[54]

IDIOPATHIC INFLAMMATORY MYOPATHIES

Idiopathic inflammatory myopathies are chronic autoimmune conditions that include juvenile dermatomyositis and juvenile polymyositis. Juvenile dermatomyositis is the most common type of inflammatory myopathy in children accounting for about 80% of cases and juvenile polymyositis is must less common accounting for 2% to 8% of cases.[56,57] The third major form of inflammatory myopathy is inclusion body myositis, but that is exceedingly rare in children. For inflammatory conditions that affect muscles, there can be different patterns of dysphagia depending on which muscles are affected and this includes tongue weakness, reduced palate and pharyngeal contractility, reduced laryngeal elevation, cricopharyngeal dysfunction, and esophageal dysmotility. The underlying pathology can be muscle atrophy or inflammatory cell invasion into the muscles and surrounding connective tissues.[58] Few publications regarding the incidence, findings, and dysphagia-related treatment outcomes focus on the pediatric population with these conditions and it is challenging to know if the adult findings can be extrapolated to children with the same conditions. Based on the EuroMyositis Registry dataset, there is a strong association with dysphagia and disease severity in idiopathic inflammatory myopathies.[59]

There are reports of successful treatment of cricopharyngeal (CP) dysfunction with CP balloon dilation,[60] botulinum toxin,[61] or myotomy[62–64] in adults with inflammatory myopathies, but there are no reports of this in the pediatric literature.

JUVENILE DERMATOMYOSITIS

In juvenile dermatomyositis, the skin and muscle are affected by capillary vasculopathy. Presentation can be as young as 13 months of age,[65] although mean age of onset is 7 years.[1] Female predilection of at least 2:1 is reported.[66–70] When males are affected, the condition may be more aggressive or present earlier.[71] Prevalence of dysphagia at presentation ranges from 15.3% to 67%.[66–74] Diagnosis is based on a muscle biopsy and if not on a diagnostic score, related to the presence of muscle weakness, skin manifestations, and laboratory measurements (anti-Jo-1 antibodies and elevated serum muscle enzymes).[75] Dysphagia results from pharyngeal weakness and/or esophageal dysmotility. Similar to scleroderma, esophageal manometry can confirm weak peristalsis of the esophageal skeletal muscle, which confirms this as cause for swallowing difficulty (**Fig. 2**).[49]

Dysphagia can be an earlier symptom in disease progression and become more common in the more severe cases of the underlying myositis[71,76] but can also be present in milder cases.[76] The presence of dysphagia portends a worse outcome from the

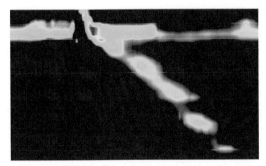

Fig. 2. Representative high-resolution esophageal manometry in a pediatric patient with juvenile dermatomyositis and dysphagia. Manometry shows a severely weakened swallow and gaps in peristalsis with ineffective esophageal motility as well as hypotensive upper and lower esophageal sphincter tone. (*From* Bayarri Moreno M, García Malagón C, Granero Cendon R, Camacho Lovillo MS, Moya Jiménez MJ. High-resolution esophageal manometry (HRM) as a potential tool for early detection of disease progression in juvenile dermatomyositis and scleroderma. An Pediatr (Engl Ed). 2024 Feb;100(2):146-147.)

underlying myositis with less likelihood to improve over time, but with treatment, dysphagia often improves.[72,77] Because reported symptoms of dysphagia do not necessarily correlate with the severity of disease and risk of aspiration, all children with active dermatomyositis should have a modified barium swallow evaluation with a speech language pathologist.[76] Treatment is primarily with high-dose corticosteroids followed by immunomodulators or other steroid-sparing agents such as IVIG and monoclonal antibodies.[66,67,69,73,75] With severe cases, supplemental enteral tube support may be indicated to support hydration and nutrition if dysphagia affects nutritional intake.

JUVENILE POLYMYOSITIS

Juvenile polymyositis is much less common compared to juvenile dermatomyositis. In contrast to dermatomyositis, the presentation of polymyositis is primarily muscle inflammation with symmetric proximal muscle weakness with an absence of skin involvement. There is at least 1 report of a case of juvenile polymyositis presenting with severe dysphagia in an adolescent.[78] There are more reports of polymyositis-associated dysphagia in the adult literature.[58,79–81]

INFECTIOUS MUCOSITIS

Acute odynophagia, dysphagia to liquids and solids, and/or prodromal symptoms of fever or chills and malaise often signal an infectious inflammatory process. Findings of oral ulcers or thrush can be clues for a pharyngeal or esophageal source of dysphagia. High suspicion for opportunistic causes of mucositis should occur in immunocompromised individuals (eg, patients with human immunodeficiency virus [HIV] or receiving chemotherapy). Other risk factors include prolonged corticosteroid use (systemic or topical) or prolonged antibiotic use.[82]

Common viral sources include herpes simplex virus and cytomegalovirus; Candida albicans is the most common fungal source; rarely, blastomycosis, aspergillosis, and histoplasmosis are other fungal sources.[83]

Diagnosis is made with endoscopic visualization and histologic confirmation of the microbial source. Neutrophilic inflammation of the tissues is typically seen surrounding the microbes under high-powered field. Tissue culture or serologic polymerization chain reaction (PCR) can also confirm the source.

Treatment is targeted at the offending microbe, with appropriate antimicrobial therapy and additional pain control such as viscous lidocaine. Intravenous therapy and rehydration can be used if oral medications are not safe or possible to take during active inflammatory response. Corticosteroids can also reduce inflammatory response, but should be used cautiously in immunosuppressed individuals.[84] More than 1 infectious source can be seen in immunocompromised patients as well. Enteral tube access can be placed during endoscopic evaluation for safe passage of nutrition, hydration, and medications. Once treated, most infectious mucositis will reduce in pain after 48 to 72 hours and completely resolve between 6 and 7 days from onset. Recurrent infection risk is higher in immunosuppressed patients, but most patients will not experience chronic dysphagia after resolution or treatment of infection.

MULTI-SYSTEM INFLAMMATORY SYNDROME DUE TO CORONAVIRUS DISEASE 2019/PEDIATRIC INFLAMMATORY MULTISYSTEM SYNDROME

Children can develop a relatively newer severe inflammatory syndrome called multi-system inflammatory syndrome due to coronavirus disease 2019 (MIS-C) or closely related pediatric inflammatory multisystem syndrome (PIMS) after a coronavirus disease 2019 (COVID-19) infection. MIS-C was first described after the onset of the pandemic as a febrile illness with laboratory evidence of systemic inflammation with multi-system involvement, including the GI tract, within 4 weeks of COVID-19 onset or exposure to the virus and no alternative diagnosis.[85] Although intubation can occur in these patients and intubation sequelae could explain the development of swallowing issues, dysphagia has been reported even in the absence of intubation. Cheong and colleagues reported that of 50 children with MIS-C at their center those who were intubated had a higher incidence of dysphagia 10/18 (56%), however, 9/32 (28%) of the non-intubated patients also developed dysphagia.[86] In a single-center study, Jenkins and colleagues found that 5 of 137 (3.6%) cases of MIS-C/PIMS developed dysphagia and that 3 of those 5 patients (60%) with dysphagia also had neck imaging identifying retropharyngeal edema or fluid collection.[87]

In the absence of intubation, there could be direct infection and inflammatory responses that affect the muscles, nervous system, and vasculature associated with swallowing.[88–90] Halfpenny and colleagues found evidence of myopathy in 2/4 (50%) of patients in their series who developed dysphagia after MIS-C/PIMS.[90] GERD may be more likely during and after the acute illness since the presence of a nasogastric tube, supine positioning, and use of sedation or paralytic agents may all increase the risk in hospitalized patients.[91] However, the exact mechanism of dysphagia and its pathophysiology due to MIS-C is not yet entirely clear.[85]

CAUSTIC INGESTION

Accidental ingestion is an emergency presentation of dysphagia and odynophagia for preschool children, with the highest risk at 3 years of age, and between 50% and 80% of all caustic ingestions occur in children.[92] When this occurs, both acidic and alkaline household products as well as button batteries can cause both a necrotic and surrounding inflammatory response to the oral cavity, oropharynx, larynx, lung, and esophagus; all of which can result in both odynophagia and dysphagia after ingestion or inhalation. Alkaline liquids cause dispersed liquefactive necrosis and inflammation, whereas acidic ingestions cause eschar formation which limits deeper tissue penetration.[93]

Early endoscopy (within 12 hours) remains the gold-standard to evaluate damage and injury to tissues. Injury can be graded by Zargar classification of severity (**Table 1**), which can guide management and predict complications.[92,94,95] Complications include acute and chronic/long-gap stricture formation, fibrosis, and altered

Table 1
Endoscopic classification of corrosive injuries according to Zarger et al[95]

Grade	Description	Endoscopy
Grade I	Edema and hyperemia of the mucosa	
Grade IIa	Superficial localized ulcerations, friability, and blisters	
Grade IIb	Circumferential and deep ulcerations	
Grade IIIa	Multiple and deep ulcerations and small scattered areas of necrosis	
Grade IIIb	Extensive necrosis	
Grade IV	Perforation	

From Cabral C, Chirica M, de Chaisemartin C, Gornet JM, Munoz-Bongrand N, Halimi B, Cattan P, Sarfati E. Caustic injuries of the upper digestive tract: a population observational study. Surg Endosc. 2012 Jan;26(1):214–221.

motility with swallowing or food impactions, and the most serious can include stenosis and fistula formation to surrounding parenchyma. Treatment for caustic tissue damage is mostly supportive, diverting nutrition by enteral tube while the tissues heal during the first several days after ingestion.[93] Esophageal treatments include serial stricture dilation with balloon dilators, and/or mitomycin C injection into damaged tissue to help tissue remodel and reduce chance for chronic stricture.[93] Long-term endoscopic surveillance is needed for secondary carcinoma risk.[93]

CONSULTATIONS

Dysphagia may be an early or presenting symptom of some acute conditions like infectious esophagitis or recent caustic ingestion or it could be a sign of more chronic or indolent conditions such as atopic or systemic autoimmune inflammatory conditions. Consultation with gastroenterology, allergy/immunology, and/or rheumatology should be considered, in-addition to otolaryngology, when there is a suspicion for an underlying systemic condition. Multidisciplinary consultation may especially be needed in the presence of other suggestive clinical manifestations such as atopy, unexplained rash, and muscle weakness or strong family history of auto-immune disease. Many children with an inflammatory cause of dysphagia are at risk for aspiration and may benefit from a modified oral diet or supportive therapies such as liquid thickeners.[16,17] An evaluation with a pediatric-trained speech language pathologist who is experienced managing dysphagia is paramount to the workup and subsequent follow-up care. Furthermore, some children may have to reduce allergen exposures or alter diets to reduce inflammatory responses and could be at risk for macro or micronutrient deficiencies after this. In these scenarios, consultation with a dietitian will assist families to meet their nutritional needs and optimize growth and development. A gastroenterologist is also integral for all patients who may need enteral nutrition with feeding tubes if they cannot fully support their diet due to swallowing deficits.

CLINICS CARE POINTS

- Maintain a high suspicion for an underlying inflammatory disorder in pediatric patients with dysphagia and suggestive clinical symptoms or signs.
- Maintain a low threshold for further testing with esophagoscopy and instrumental swallow studies when an underlying inflammatory disorder is present or suspected because some patients can present with minimal or non-specific symptoms but have treatable pathology on diagnostic testing.
- Evaluation should include a speech language pathology consultation to fully assess the dysphagia that may be multi-factorial.
- Management is often multi-disciplinary.

DISCLOSURE

The authors have nothing to disclose.

REFERENCES

1. Nelson SP, Chen EH, Syniar GM, et al. Prevalence of symptoms of gastroesophageal reflux during infancy. A pediatric practice-based survey. Pediatric Practice Research Group. Arch Pediatr Adolesc Med 1997;151(6):569–72.

2. Hassall E. Decisions in diagnosing and managing chronic gastroesophageal reflux disease in children. J Pediatr 2005;146(3 Supplement):S3–12.

3. Mousa H, Hassan M. Gastroesophageal reflux disease. Pediatr Clin North Am 2017;64(3):487–505.

4. Rosen R, Vandenplas Y, Singendonk M, et al. Pediatric gastroesophageal reflux clinical practice guidelines: joint recommendations of the North American Society for pediatric gastroenterology, hepatology, and nutrition and the european society for pediatric gastroenterology, hepatology, and nutrition. J Pediatr Gastroenterol Nutr 2018;66(3):516–54.

5. Pearson EG, Downey EC, Barnhart DC, et al. Reflux esophageal stricture–a review of 30 years' experience in children. J Pediatr Surg 2010;45(12):2356–60.

6. Vandenplas Y. Management of benign esophageal strictures in children. Pediatr Gastroenterol Hepatol Nutr 2017;20(4):211–5.

7. Sohouli MH, Alimadadi H, Rohani P, et al. Esophageal stents for the management of benign esophageal strictures in children and adolescents: a systematic review of observational studies. Dysphagia 2023;38(3):744–55.

8. Ferenczy JJ, Glenn JB. Total obliteration and subsequent recanalization of esophagus via endoscopic rendezvous procedure in a pediatric patient. Am Surg 2022; 88(9):2198–9.

9. Slater BJ, Rothenberg SS. Fundoplication. Clin Perinatol 2017;44(4):795–803.

10. King M, Barnhart DC, O'Gorman M, et al. Effect of gastrojejunal feedings on visits and costs in children with neurologic impairment. J Pediatr Gastroenterol Nutr 2014;58(4):518–24.

11. Koufman JA, Aviv JE, Casiano RR, et al. Laryngopharyngeal reflux: position statement of the committee on speech, voice, and swallowing disorders of the American Academy of Otolaryngology-Head and Neck Surgery. Otolaryngol Head Neck Surg 2002;127(1):32–5.

12. Orenstein SR. An overview of reflux-associated disorders in infants: apnea, laryngospasm, and aspiration. Am J Med 2001;111(Suppl 8A):60S–3S.

13. Zalesska-Krecicka M, Krecicki T, Iwanczak B, et al. Laryngeal manifestations of gastroesophageal reflux disease in children. Acta Otolaryngol 2002;122(3): 306–10.

14. Aviv JE, Liu H, Parides M, et al. Laryngopharyngeal sensory deficits in patients with laryngopharyngeal reflux and dysphagia. Ann Otol Rhinol Laryngol 2000; 109(11):1000–6.

15. Thompson DM. Laryngopharyngeal sensory testing and assessment of airway protection in pediatric patients. Am J Med 2003;115(Suppl 3A):166S–8S.

16. Suskind DL, Thompson DM, Gulati M, et al. Improved infant swallowing after gastroesophageal reflux disease treatment: a function of improved laryngeal sensation? Laryngoscope 2006;116(8):1397–403.

17. Rossoni EP, Miranda VSG, Barbosa LDR. The prevalence of dysphagia in children with laryngomalacia pre and postsupraglottoplasty: a systematic review with meta-analysis. Int Arch Otorhinolaryngol 2024;28(1):e170–6.

18. Luebke K, Samuels TL, Chelius TH, et al. Pepsin as a biomarker for laryngopharyngeal reflux in children with laryngomalacia. Laryngoscope 2017;127(10): 2413–7.

19. Iyer VK, Pearman K, Raafat F. Laryngeal mucosal histology in laryngomalacia: the evidence for gastro-oesophageal reflux laryngitis. Int J Pediatr Otorhinolaryngol 1999;49(3):225–30.

20. Powitzky R, Stoner J, Fisher T, et al. Changes in sleep apnea after supraglotto-plasty in infants with laryngomalacia. Int J Pediatr Otorhinolaryngol 2011; 75(10):1234–9.
21. Rastatter JC, Schroeder JW, Hoff SR, et al. Aspiration before and after Supraglot-toplasty regardless of Technique. Int J Otolaryngol 2010;2010:912814.
22. Duncan DR, Larson K, Davidson K, et al. Acid suppression does not improve lar-yngomalacia outcomes but treatment for oropharyngeal dysphagia might be pro-tective. J Pediatr 2021;238:42–9.e2.
23. Apps JR, Flint JD, Wacogne I. Towards evidence based medicine for paediatri-cians. Question 1. Does anti-reflux therapy improve symptoms in infants with lar-yngomalacia? Arch Dis Child 2012;97(4):385–7, discussion 387.
24. Hartl TT, Chadha NK. A systematic review of laryngomalacia and acid reflux. Oto-laryngol Head Neck Surg 2012;147(4):619–26.
25. Landres RT, Kuster GG, Strum WB. Eosinophilic esophagitis in a patient with vigorous achalasia. Gastroenterology 1978;74(6):1298–301.
26. Robson J, O'Gorman M, McClain A, et al. Incidence and prevalence of pediatric eosinophilic esophagitis in utah based on a 5-year population-based study. Clin Gastroenterol 2019;17(1):107–14.e1.
27. Dellon ES, Jensen ET, Martin CF, et al. Prevalence of eosinophilic esophagitis in the United States. Clin Gastroenterol 2014;12(4):589–96.e1.
28. Kia L, Hirano I. Advances in the endoscopic evaluation of eosinophilic esophagi-tis. Curr Opin Gastroenterol 2016;32(4):325–31.
29. Furuta GT, Katzka DA. Eosinophilic esophagitis. N Engl J Med 2015;373(17): 1640–8.
30. Menard-Katcher C, Swerdlow MP, Mehta P, et al. Contribution of esophagram to the evaluation of complicated pediatric eosinophilic esophagitis. J Pediatr Gas-troenterol Nutr 2015;61(5):541–6.
31. Spergel JM. Eosinophilic esophagitis in adults and children: evidence for a food allergy component in many patients. Curr Opin Allergy Clin Immunol 2007;7(3): 274–8.
32. Yawn RJ, Acra S, Goudy SL, et al. Eosinophilic laryngitis in children with aerodi-gestive dysfunction. Otolaryngol–Head Neck 2015;153(1):124–9.
33. Smith LP, Chewaproug L, Spergel JM, et al. Otolaryngologists may not be doing enough to diagnose pediatric eosinophilic esophagitis. Int J Pediatr Otorhinolar-yngol 2009;73(11):1554–7.
34. Dauer EH, Freese DK, El-Youssef M, et al. Clinical characteristics of eosinophilic esophagitis in children. Ann Otol Rhinol Laryngol 2005;114(11):827–33.
35. Rubio CA, Sjödahl K, Lagergren J. Lymphocytic esophagitis: a histologic subset of chronic esophagitis. Am J Clin Pathol 2006;125(3):432–7.
36. Purdy JK, Appelman HD, Golembeski CP, et al. Lymphocytic esophagitis: a chronic or recurring pattern of esophagitis resembling allergic contact dermatitis. Am J Clin Pathol 2008;130(4):508–13.
37. Rouphael C, Gordon IO, Thota PN. Lymphocytic esophagitis: Still an enigma a decade later. World J Gastroenterol 2017;23(6):949–56.
38. Sutton LM, Heintz DD, Patel AS, et al. Lymphocytic esophagitis in children. In-flamm Bowel Dis 2014;20(8):1324–8.
39. Lauritano D, Boccalari E, Di Stasio D, et al. Prevalence of oral lesions and corre-lation with intestinal symptoms of inflammatory bowel disease: a systematic re-view. Diagn Basel Switz 2019;9(3):77.
40. Ramaswamy K, Jacobson K, Jevon G, et al. Esophageal crohn disease in chil-dren: a clinical spectrum. J Pediatr Gastroenterol Nutr 2003;36(4):454–8.

41. Ammoury RF, Pfefferkorn MD. Significance of esophageal Crohn disease in children. J Pediatr Gastroenterol Nutr 2011;52(3):291–4.
42. Vale Rodrigues R, Sladek M, Katsanos K, et al. Diagnosis and outcome of oesophageal crohn's disease. J Crohns Colitis 2020;14(5):624–9.
43. Li SC. Scleroderma in children and adolescents: localized scleroderma and systemic sclerosis. Pediatr Clin North Am 2018;65(4):757–81.
44. Misra R, Singh G, Aggarwal P, et al. Juvenile onset systemic sclerosis: a single center experience of 23 cases from Asia. Clin Rheumatol 2007;26(8):1259–62.
45. Donzelli G, Carnesecchi G, Amador C, et al. Fetal programming and systemic sclerosis. Am J Obstet Gynecol 2015;213(6):839.e1–8.
46. Rutkowska-Sak L, Gietka P, Gazda A, et al. Juvenile systemic sclerosis - observations of one clinical centre. Reumatologia 2021;59(6):367–72.
47. Frati Munari AC, Culebro Nieves G, Velázquez E, et al. [Scleroderma in children]. Bol Med Hosp Infant Mex 1979;36(2):201–14.
48. van den Hoogen F, Khanna D, Fransen J, et al. 2013 classification criteria for systemic sclerosis: an American college of rheumatology/European league against rheumatism collaborative initiative. Ann Rheum Dis 2013;72(11):1747–55.
49. Bayarri Moreno M, García Malagón C, Granero Cendon R, et al. High-resolution esophageal manometry (HRM) as a potential tool for early detection of disease progression in juvenile dermatomyositis and scleroderma. An Pediatr 2024; 100(2):146–7.
50. Valões CCM, Novak GV, Brunelli JB, et al. Esophageal abnormalities in juvenile localized scleroderma: is it associated with other extracutaneous manifestations? Rev Bras Reumatol 2017;57(6):521–5.
51. Weber P, Ganser G, Frosch M, et al. Twenty-four hour intraesophageal pH monitoring in children and adolescents with scleroderma and mixed connective tissue disease. J Rheumatol 2000;27(11):2692–5.
52. Guariso G, Conte S, Galeazzi F, et al. Esophageal involvement in juvenile localized scleroderma: a pilot study. Clin Exp Rheumatol 2007;25(5):786–9.
53. Luebker S, Frech TM, Assassi S, et al. The Collaborative National Quality and Efficacy Registry for Scleroderma: association of medication use on gastrointestinal tract symptoms in early disease and the importance of tobacco cessation. Clin Exp Rheumatol 2023;41(8):1632–8.
54. Vivino FB, Bunya VY, Massaro-Giordano G, et al. Sjogren's syndrome: An update on disease pathogenesis, clinical manifestations and treatment. Clin Immunol Orlando Fla 2019;203:81–121.
55. De Oliveira MA, De Rezende NPM, Maia CMF, et al. Primary Sjögren syndrome in a 2-year-old patient: role of the dentist in diagnosis and dental management with a 6-year follow-up. Int J Paediatr Dent 2011;21(6):471–5.
56. Feldman BM, Rider LG, Reed AM, et al. Juvenile dermatomyositis and other idiopathic inflammatory myopathies of childhood. Lancet Lond Engl 2008;371(9631): 2201–12.
57. Shah M, Mamyrova G, Targoff IN, et al. The clinical phenotypes of the juvenile idiopathic inflammatory myopathies. Medicine (Baltimore) 2013;92(1):25–41.
58. Kagen LJ, Hochman RB, Strong EW. Cricopharyngeal obstruction in inflammatory myopathy (polymyositis/dermatomyositis). report of three cases and review of the literature. Arthritis Rheum 1985;28(6):630–6.
59. Lilleker JB, Vencovsky J, Wang G, et al. The EuroMyositis registry: an international collaborative tool to facilitate myositis research. Ann Rheum Dis 2018; 77(1):30–9.

60. Nagano H, Yoshifuku K, Kurono Y. Polymyositis with dysphagia treated with endoscopic balloon dilatation. Auris Nasus Larynx 2009;36(6):705–8.

61. Liu LWC, Tarnopolsky M, Armstrong D. Injection of botulinum toxin A to the upper esophageal sphincter for oropharyngeal dysphagia in two patients with inclusion body myositis. Can J Gastroenterol J Can Gastroenterol 2004;18(6):397–9.

62. Riminton DS, Chambers ST, Parkin PJ, et al. Inclusion body myositis presenting solely as dysphagia. Neurology 1993;43(6):1241–3.

63. Vencovský J, Rehák F, Pafko P, et al. Acute cricopharyngeal obstruction in dermatomyositis. J Rheumatol 1988;15(6):1016–8.

64. Bachmann G, Streppel M, Krug B, et al. Cricopharyngeal muscle hypertrophy associated with florid myositis. Dysphagia 2001;16(4):244–8.

65. Rachadi H, Bouayad K, Chiheb S. [Juvenile dermatomyositis: early onset and unusual presentation]. Arch Pediatr Organe 2016;23(10):1071–5.

66. Cancarini P, Nozawa T, Whitney K, et al. The clinical features of juvenile dermatomyositis: A single-centre inception cohort. Semin Arthritis Rheum 2022;57: 152104.

67. Simmons E, Kazmi M, Wilson M, et al. Characteristics of patients with juvenile dermatomyositis from 2001-2021 at a tertiary care center. Dermatol Online J 2022; 28(6). https://doi.org/10.5070/D328659719.

68. Sarkar S, Mondal T, Saha A, et al. Profile of pediatric idiopathic inflammatory myopathies from a tertiary care center of Eastern India. Indian J Pediatr 2017;84(4): 299–306.

69. Al-Mayouf SM, AlMutiari N, Muzaffer M, et al. Phenotypic characteristics and outcome of juvenile dermatomyositis in Arab children. Rheumatol Int 2017; 37(9):1513–7.

70. Chiu SK, Yang YH, Wang LC, et al. Ten-year experience of juvenile dermatomyositis: a retrospective study. J Microbiol Immunol Infect Wei Mian Yu Gan Ran Za Zhi 2007;40(1):68–73.

71. Felix A, Delion F, Louis-Sidney F, et al. Juvenile dermatomyositis in afro-caribbean children: a cohort study in the french west indies. Pediatr Rheumatol Online J 2023;21(1):113.

72. Chickermane PR, Mankad D, Khubchandani RP. Disease patterns of juvenile dermatomyositis from Western India. Indian Pediatr 2013;50(10):961–3.

73. Prasad S, Misra R, Agarwal V, et al. Juvenile dermatomyositis at a tertiary care hospital: is there any change in the last decade? Int J Rheum Dis 2013;16(5): 556–60.

74. Pachman LM, Morgan G, Klein-Gitelman MS, et al. Nailfold capillary density in 140 untreated children with juvenile dermatomyositis: an indicator of disease activity. Pediatr Rheumatol Online J 2023;21(1):118.

75. Leung AKC, Lam JM, Alobaida S, et al. Juvenile dermatomyositis: advances in pathogenesis, assessment, and management. Curr Pediatr Rev 2021;17(4): 273–87.

76. McCann LJ, Garay SM, Ryan MM, et al. Oropharyngeal dysphagia in juvenile dermatomyositis (JDM): an evaluation of videofluoroscopy swallow study (VFSS) changes in relation to clinical symptoms and objective muscle scores. Rheumatol Oxf Engl 2007;46(8):1363–6.

77. Challa D, Crowson CS, Niewold TB, et al, CARRA Legacy Registry Investigators. Predictors of changes in disease activity among children with juvenile dermatomyositis enrolled in the Childhood Arthritis and Rheumatology Research Alliance (CARRA) Legacy Registry. Clin Rheumatol 2018;37(4):1011–5.

78. Patel R, Zala U, Chaudhari J, et al. An unusual presentation of juvenile polymyositis in an adolescent girl. Cureus 2023;15(1):e33249.

79. Cavazzana I, Fredi M, Selmi C, et al. The clinical and histological spectrum of idiopathic inflammatory myopathies. Clin Rev Allergy Immunol 2017;52(1):88–98.

80. de Merieux P, Verity MA, Clements PJ, et al. Esophageal abnormalities and dysphagia in polymyositis and dermatomyositis. Arthritis Rheum 1983;26(8): 961–8.

81. Jacob H, Berkowitz D, McDonald E, et al. The esophageal motility disorder of polymyositis. a prospective study. Arch Intern Med 1983;143(12):2262–4.

82. Bordea MA, Pîrvan A, Gheban D, et al. Infectious esophagitis in romanian children: from etiology and risk factors to clinical characteristics and endoscopic features. J Clin Med 2020;9(4). https://doi.org/10.3390/jcm9040939.

83. Flasar M, Raufman JP. Esophageal infections. In: Schlossberg D, editor. *Clinical infectious disease*. 2nd edition. Cambridge, UK: Cambridge University Press; 2015. p. 324–33.

84. Rosołowski M, Kierzkiewicz M. Etiology, diagnosis and treatment of infectious esophagitis. Przeglad Gastroenterol 2013;8(6):333–7.

85. Tutor JD. COVID-19 and Dysphagia in Children: A Review. Dysphagia 2023; 38(1):122–6.

86. Cheong RCT, Jephson C, Frauenfelder C, et al. Otolaryngologic Manifestations in Pediatric Inflammatory Multisystem Syndrome Temporally Associated With COVID-19. JAMA Otolaryngol– Head Neck Surg 2021;147(5):482–4.

87. Jenkins E, Sherry W, Smith AGC, et al. Retropharyngeal Edema and Neck Pain in Multisystem Inflammatory Syndrome in Children (MIS-c). J Pediatr Infect Dis Soc 2021;10(9):922–5.

88. Lin JE, Asfour A, Sewell TB, et al. Neurological issues in children with COVID-19. Neurosci Lett 2021;743:135567.

89. Song E, Zhang C, Israelow B, et al. Neuroinvasion of SARS-CoV-2 in human and mouse brain. J Exp Med 2021;218(3). https://doi.org/10.1084/jem.20202135.

90. Halfpenny R, Stewart A, Carter A, et al. Dysphonia and dysphagia consequences of paediatric inflammatory multisystem syndrome temporally associated with SARS-CoV-2 (PIMS-TS). Int J Pediatr Otorhinolaryngol 2021;148:110823.

91. Macht M, Wimbish T, Bodine C, et al. ICU-acquired swallowing disorders. Crit Care Med 2013;41(10):2396–405.

92. Bonavina L, Chirica M, Skrobic O, et al. Foregut caustic injuries: results of the world society of emergency surgery consensus conference. World J Emerg Surg WJES 2015;10:44.

93. Arnold M, Numanoglu A. Caustic ingestion in children-A review. Semin Pediatr Surg 2017;26(2):95–104.

94. Cabral C, Chirica M, de Chaisemartin C, et al. Caustic injuries of the upper digestive tract: a population observational study. Surg Endosc 2012;26(1):214–21.

95. Zargar SA, Kochhar R, Mehta S, et al. The role of fiberoptic endoscopy in the management of corrosive ingestion and modified endoscopic classification of burns. Gastrointest Endosc 1991;37(2):165–9.

Dysphagia in the Aging Population

Courtney J. Hunter, MD[a], Ozlem E. Tulunay-Ugur, MD[b],*

KEYWORDS

- Dysphagia • Elderly • Geriatric • Presbyphagia • Swallowing disorder

KEY POINTS

- The aging population has unique physiologic changes that contribute to dysphagia, which perpetuates declining health. Namely, sarcopenia, which is the age-related decline in muscle mass, is a primary contributing factor.
- The aging population is especially susceptible to neurologic, musculoskeletal, pulmonary, and nutritional decline, which only compounds the effects of dysphagia.
- The authors advocate for a patient-centered approach to dysphagia management in the aging population with goals of care outlines and open multidisciplinary communication.

INTRODUCTION

Dysphagia is defined as having difficulty with swallowing, which may include patients with changes related to chewing, swallowing, or transit of the food distally to the stomach.[1] Approximately 300,000 to 600,000 United States (US) patients are affected by dysphagia annually, with 15% to 30% of adults over 65 years-old estimated to have dysphagia, even this is likely a gross underestimation.[2,3] Relatedly, 70% of all dysphagia referrals represent patients over the age of 60, which is of particular importance when considering the World's aging population.[2,4] The 2020 US Census[5] saw its greatest growth rate in elderly population density since the late 19th century: from 13% to 16.8% of the total population. As the population continues to age, it is paramount to understand the physiologic changes that accompany aging, to be able to appropriately manage this growing group of future patients.

[a] Department of Otolaryngology-Head and Neck Surgery, University of Arkansas for Medical Sciences, 4301 W. Markham Street, Slot 543, Little Rock, AR 72205, USA; [b] Division of Laryngology, University of Arkansas for Medical Sciences, 4301 W. Markham Street, Slot 543, Little Rock, AR 72205, USA
* Corresponding author. Patricia and J. Floyd Kyser, MD Professor in Otolaryngology Head and Neck Surgery, Director, Division of Laryngology, University of Arkansas for Medical Sciences, Little Rock, AR 72205.
E-mail address: oetulunayugur@uams.edu

Otolaryngol Clin N Am 57 (2024) 685–693
https://doi.org/10.1016/j.otc.2024.03.006
0030-6665/24/© 2024 Elsevier Inc. All rights reserved.

DISCUSSION
Effects of Aging on Swallowing

The process of a safe and efficient swallow is complicated at baseline, and the swallowing process can be influenced by all of the factors mentioned in previous articles. The authors aim to discuss how each phase of swallowing can be susceptible to the effects of aging–presbyphagia.[6] Few articles have demonstrated before that even in the healthy older adult, changes are to be expected, as only 16% demonstrated a completely normal swallow on videofluoroscopy, with pharyngeal residue being the most common abnormality.[7]

Oral phase changes

The food bolus is often immature because of changes in mechanical and sensory processing. Cognitive processing of textures, volume, taste, and temperature of the food bolus can be diminished.[6] Additionally, loss of dentition that leads to reduced mechanical efficiency by up to 50% prolongs the length of time; the food bolus remains in the oral cavity in addition to limiting food choices.[6] Other notable changes of aging include decrease in the cross-sectional area of the muscles of mastication leading to weaker mastication, as well as decreased salivary production resulting in limited enzyme production and poor dentition. Decreased muscle bulk, range of motion of the connective tissues, and sensation of the oropharynx can change the rate of delivery of the bolus to the pharynx.[6] Premature spillage into the pharynx and delivery of the bolus during inspiratory phase can lead to pre-swallowing aspiration.[8]

Pharyngeal phase changes

Pharyngeal constrictor muscles that narrow to propel the bolus from the oropharynx through the upper esophageal sphincter (UES) weaken with aging, leading to weaker propulsion into the esophagus. Similarly, hyolaryngeal elevation is slower in older adults because of decreased tissue elasticity and a lower sitting larynx.[9] Therefore, the larynx will often not have completely reached its full range of motion before the bolus passes, hence, increasing the risk of aspiration. The incomplete elevation of the larynx furthermore limits the opening of the UES itself, significantly compounding dysphagia.[10] Delayed and incomplete relaxation of the cricopharyngeal (CP) muscle allows for the food bolus to pool in the pyriform sinuses.[11] The decreased compliance of the UES further slows the swallow and increases the risk of pharyngeal stasis and subsequent aspiration.[11]

Esophageal phase changes

Generalized weakness of the esophagus is more common in the aging adult with lower density of striated muscle in the proximal esophagus, tertiary contractions, and frank aperistalsis.[11,12] Decreased amplitude of esophageal contractions is prevalent in patients above the age of 80.[11] A slower esophageal transit has been associated with higher sensory thresholds because of nerve degeneration.[11,12]

Systems Complicating Dysphagia in the Elderly

Neurologic

Perhaps the most salient system affected by aging is the neurologic system. At the cellular level, the aging process effects chemical transmission and neurologic communication via decreased nerve velocity and sensory processing resulting in neurodegredation.[6] Blood flow is also decreased as dedicated MRI studies have shown slower cerebral blood flow and smaller volume cerebral nuclei in the elderly population.[13] Similarly, slower neurologic coordination of swallowing because of slower afferent sensory signal transmission leading to slower pharyngeal response to a food bolus have been associated with advanced age.[11,14,15] All of the afore-mentioned processes contribute to baseline neurologic dysphagia in the aging population.

Moreover, neurologic insults can exacerbate these baseline swallowing difficulties further. It is estimated that 400,000 to 500,000 people are affected by a stroke in the US annually, and this number is expected to increase with the aging population.[16] Immediately following a stroke, approximately half of patients experience oropharyn-geal dysphagia—predominantly silent aspiration.[2,11,17,18] Acute stroke dysphagia is related to altered mental status, generalized weakness, and dyscoordination.[2,19] Many stroke victims will return to their baseline swallowing function within 1 month of the stroke, but others will have persistent dysphagia in the long-term.[17]

Aging adults with neurodegenerative diseases also bear special consideration. Neurodegenerative diseases traditionally have multiple bulbar weaknesses contrib-uting to dysphagia but can also include patients with progressive dementia. Dementia and mild cognitive impairment have a prevalence of 10% and 22% among the elderly population, respectively.[20] Nearly half of patients with dementia have dysphagia most commonly because of the slowing of the swallowing process.[21] The degree of dysphagia is exacerbated by cognitive impairment and decreased appetite. Other degenerative diseases of the central nervous system, including amyotrophic lateral sclerosis (ALS), multiple sclerosis, and Parkinson's disease, have similar manifesta-tions of dysphagia..[22] While ALS is associated with delayed swallow reflex and hyper-tonia of the UES, Parkinson's disease can lead to lingual tremor, delayed oral transit times, as well as glottic insufficiency resulting in higher risk of aspiration.[11,23]

Musculoskeletal strength

Sarcopenic dysphagia is decline in swallowing, related to the progressive loss of total body muscle mass.[1] Sarcopenia frequently begins in the fifth decade of life, affecting approximately 10% to 40% of people in this age group.[24] The progressive weakness and decreased muscle mass limits the flexibility of tendons and coordination of mus-cle groups. The small muscles required for an efficient and safe swallow are easily affected. This can contribute to decreased thickness of the tongue and geniohyoid muscles, causing weaker tongue pressure and pharyngeal muscle contraction.[25–27] Additionally, cartilaginous structures mature with age limiting their functional elasticity contributing to loss of range of motion leading to decreased laryngeal elevation and wider pharyngeal diameter during swallow.[2,26]

A study of patients with clinical sarcopenia without symptoms of dysphagia showed increased EAT-10 scores and swallowing time, indicating early evidence of swallowing dysfunction.[28] Similarly, swallowing safety has been directly associated with upper arm circumference, which is generally accepted as a reliable measure of sarcopenia.[29]

Impaired mastication, poor dentition, and pain with chewing, may lead to food avoidance, further perpetuating sarcopenia.[1] Fiber, fruits, and raw vegetables are particularly difficult to chew, thus avoided, contributing to malnutrition.[30] Patients with impaired mastication opt for softer, nutrient depleted foods such as potatoes and breads intensifying the decline.[31]

Pulmonary clearance

True vocal fold atrophy because of aging can lead to glottic insufficiency, rendering patients susceptible to aspiration. Glottic incompetence leading to an ineffective coughing can increase the patient's risk of aspiration pneumonia, as well as asphyx-iation and death. Decreased pulmonary function and clearance make aspiration events more dangerous because of inability to clear tracheal and bronchial contents.[6]

Aging is associated with reduced lung compliance and impaired mucociliary clearance, thus, making the lungs more susceptible to insults.[32]

Polypharmacy

Older patients tend to have multiple comorbid conditions that are being treated by different providers. More than 33% of patients over the age of 65 are prescribed 5 or more prescription medications.[33,34] Furthermore, more than 66% of older adults take over the counter and self-prescribed supplements in addition to their prescription medications.[34] Older patients are more sensitive to the sedating properties of medications, which can impair swallowing, as well as cough reflexes.[35] A common side effect of medications such as antihypertensives, proton pump inhibitors, anticholinergics, and antidepressants is xerostomia.[33] Adequate saliva production is important for oral enzymatic digestion of food, lubrication of food during swallow, and overall dental health. Xerostomia has been associated with decreased quality of life (QoL) outcomes.[36]

Mechanical or functional obstruction

Various pathologies lead to oropharyngeal dysphagia in the older population. Patients characteristically describe food "sticking" in the neck, which can be caused by anatomic changes. One such pathology is UES dysfunction or CP dysfunction, which is associated with increased thickness or tone of the circular CP musculature contributing to incomplete opening of the UES.[11] Other pathologies include cervical spine osteophytes, most commonly between C5 andC7, projecting anteriorly leading to posterior pharyngeal wall ledge causing solid food dysphagia [37]; and Zenker's diverticulum resulting in solid food dysphagia, as well as regurgitation, aspiration, and weight loss.[11] Head and neck malignancy as a cause of dysphagia must also be ruled out, especially in the chronic tobacco or alcohol users.

Complications of Dysphagia

Dysphagia, especially in the elderly, has multiple grave health implications including malnutrition, aspiration pneumonia, and asphyxiation—all possibly contributing to death.[14,38]

Malnutrition

Nutritional status is the cornerstone and indicator of overall health. Poor nutritional status contributes to muscle mass loss and expediting sarcopenia.[1,39] Dysphagia and factors such as stress, restrictions in mobility, social factors, and limited access to healthcare, all contribute to malnutrition.[1] It is estimated that between 6% to 30% of older persons are malnourished, and this number is higher in the acute setting.[40] Severity of malnutrition general nutrition status can be easily quantified with Mini-Nutritional Assessment Short-Form and serum albumin levels.[1] Malnutrition inhibits the body's innate defense mechanisms and worsens the effects of both acute and chronic illnesses. Malnutrition is considered one of the main modifiable risk factors for poor outcomes in older patients.[1] In a never-ending cycle, malnutrition, poor oral health, sarcopenia, and dysphagia will continue to compound their effects and contribute to overall frailty.

Aspiration pneumonia

Patients above the age of 75 years are 6 times more likely to suffer from aspiration pneumonia, compared with their younger counterparts.[22] The increased incidence of pneumonia with aging has been associated with impaired cough reflex because of hypoesthesia of the supraglottic tissues, among other changes such as slow pharyngeal transit time, decreased hyolaryngeal excursion, delayed laryngeal vestibule closure, and poor UES opening.[6,22,41]

As a result of decreased salivary clearance, oral flora colonization with *Staphylococcus aureus*, *Klebsiella pneumoniae* and *Escherichia coli* is more common.[42–44] Aspiration of these pathogens can be perilous, especially, with innate immune system declines associated with aging.

Aspiration pneumonia is especially prevalent in the post-stroke patient population because of the acute functional neurologic insult. A reported 10% to 30% of post-stroke patients have persistent dysphagia with aspiration.[45] Aspiration pneumonia can affect up to one-third of acute stroke patients and contributes to 35% of post-stroke deaths.[46]

MANAGEMENT OF DYSPHAGIA
Timing and Interventions

Management of dysphagia requires a multidisciplinary, patient centered approach. The management is complex because of lack of concise guidelines, as well as each patient presenting with varying needs, goals of care, complex medical histories, and frailty. The dysphagia team should include primary care providers/geriatricians, speech, and language pathologists, otolaryngologists, dieticians, physical and occupational therapists, neurologists, ethicists, family members, and pulmonologists.

Video fluoroscopic swallow study is the mainstay of diagnosis and management in patients with dysphagia. It also helps to identify areas for intervention. Work-up starts with indirect laryngostroboscopy to rule out masses or lesions; to assess true vocal fold movement; glottic sufficiency; and vallecular and pharyngeal residue (**Fig. 1**). Swallowing therapy and diet modifications are the cornerstone of management.

Cervical spine osteophytes may present with dysphagia in about 10% of dysphagic patients.[11] Treatment of dysphagia in these cases is predominantly managed with diet

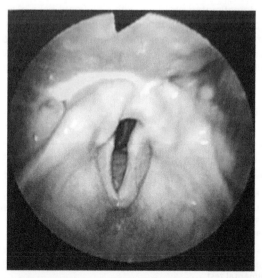

Fig. 1. Bilateral vocal fold paralysis identified on indirect laryngoscopy with bilateral vocal folds fixed in a paramedian position with bowing with evidence of pharyngeal pooling and frank aspiration.

modifications. If the clinical manifestation of dysphagia is severe, patients can be referred to spine surgeon for excision of the osteophyte.

Zenker's diverticulum can be managed with observation, whereas larger and more symptomatic diverticulums require surgical intervention. Symptoms requiring intervention include malnutrition, weight loss, regurgitation of food, and aspiration.[11] Management of the diverticulum depends on surgeon preference, as well as patient factors. Many patients can be managed with an endoscopic approach with division of the common wall with carbon dioxide laser or gastric stapler.[11] If exposure with diverticuloscope is difficult due to neck extension or location of the diverticulum, open diverticulectomy can be performed via transcervical approach.

CP muscle dysfunction is one of the most common anatomic sources of dysphagia in the elderly population—primarily presenting as solid food dysphagia.[47] Management of CP muscle dysfunction includes diet modification, botulinum toxin injection, dilation, and CP myotomy.[48] Similar to other interventions mentioned before, decisions to escalate treatment depend on the severity of patient symptoms and response to prior treatments. After failing diet modifications, CP dilation with balloon of 18 to 20 mm may be pursued.[11] A more unique approach to dilation is gaining popularity using 2 balloons of 15 mm side by side in the esophageal inlet to gain an even more robust result.[49]

Gastrostomy tube feeding should be reserved for patients who have exhausted all other interventions for advanced dysphagia, and who are significantly malnourished or at risk for aspiration. Patients with neurodegenerative diseases with progressive dysphagia (ie, dementia and Alzheimer's disease) may require enteral access because of discoordination of swallowing and decreased appetite. It is important to note that the presence of gastrostomy tube is not associated with decreased rates of aspiration pneumonia or increased rates of survival.[50] The authors advocate for a discussion between the patient, family members, and providers early in diagnosis to determine the patient's wishes for non-oral means of nutrition.

SUMMARY

Dysphagia is an underestimated problem, with significant risks of morbidity and mortality, for the older person. It is compounded by sarcopenia, polypharmacy, and physiologic changes of aging. Dysphagia in the elderly leads to considerable reduction inQoL and social isolation. Hence, the job of the otolaryngologist is not only to manage dysphagia surgically, but also to help patients and caregivers navigate medical decisions and ethical choices.

CLINICS CARE POINTS

- Dysphagia in the elderly can lead to malnutrition, dehydration, asphyxiation, and death.
- There are many physiologic changes in the swallowing system because of aging.
- Sarcopenia, which is loss of muscle mass, exacerbates the aging changes of the swallowing system. The resultant dysphagia in turn increases sarcopenia. Therefore, when treating patients, special attention needs to be paid to the nutritional status, degree of sarcopenia, and degree of frailty.
- Many methods exist to assess nutritional status and degree of frailty, which can be adapted as part of routine practice. These include prealbumin levels, grip strength, walk-up-and-go test, EAT-10, minimental test.
- Common pathologies of aging are CP dysfunction and Zenker's diverticulum. Otolaryngologists should familiarize themselves with multiple techniques to manage these.

• Dysphagia management is a team effort; institutions should invest in personalized dysphagia care and more importantly early detection and collaborative management.

DISCLOSURE

The authors have nothing to disclose.

REFERENCES

1. de Sire A, Ferrillo M, Lippi L, et al. Sarcopenic Dysphagia, Malnutrition, and Oral Frailty in Elderly: A Comprehensive Review. Nutrients 2022;14(5):982.
2. Sura L, Madhavan A, Carnaby G, et al. Dysphagia in the elderly: management and nutritional considerations. Clin Interv Aging 2012;7:287–98.
3. Barczi SR, Sullivan PA, Robbins J. How should dysphagia care of older adults differ? Establishing optimal practice patterns. Semin Speech Lang 2000;21:347–61.
4. Leder SB, Suiter D. An epidemiologic study on aging and dysphagia in the acute care hospitalized population: 2000-2007. Gerontology 2009;55:714–8.
5. U.S. Census Bureau. The older population: 2020. Available at: https://www.census.gov/library/publications/2023/decennial/c2020br-07.html#:~:text=The%20older%20population%20in%20the,the%20total%20population%20in%202020. [Accessed 20 December 2023].
6. Feng HY, Zhang PP, Wang XW. Presbyphagia: Dysphagia in the elderly. World J Clin Cases 2023;11(11):2363–73.
7. Ekberg O, Feinberg MJ. Altered swallowing function in elderly patients without dysphagia: radiologic findings in 56 cases. AJR Am J Roentgenol 1991;156:1181–4.
8. Ortega O, Martín A, Clavé P. Diagnosis and Management of Oropharyngeal Dysphagia Among Older Persons, State of the Art. J Am Med Dir Assoc 2017;18:576–82.
9. Yokoyama M, Mitomi N, Tetsuka K, et al. Role of laryngeal movement and effect of aging on swallowing pressure in the pharynx and upper esophageal sphincter. Laryngoscope 2000;110:434–9.
10. Kletzien H, Cullins MJ, Connor NP. Age-related alterations in swallowing biomechanics. Exp Gerontol 2019;118:45–50.
11. Achem SR, DeVault KR. Dysphagia in Aging. J Clin Gastroenterol 2005;39(5):357–71.
12. Meshkinpour H, Haghighat P, Dutton C. Clinical spectrum of esophageal aperistalsis in the elderly. Am J Gastroenterol 1994;89:1480–3.
13. Bertoni-Freddari C, Fattoretti P, Paoloni R, et al. Synaptic structural dynamics and aging. Gerontology 1996;42:170–80.
14. Mehraban-Far S, Alrassi J, Patel R, et al. Dysphagia in the elderly population: A videofluoroscopic study. American Journal of Otolaryngology-Haed and Neck Medicine and Surgery 2021;42:102854.
15. Koton S, Sang Y, Schneider ALC, et al. Trends in Stroke Incidence Rates in Older US Adults: An Update from the Atherosclerosis Risk in Communities (ARIC) Cohort Study. JAMA Neurol 2020;77(1):109–13.
16. American Heart Association. 1992 heart and stroke facts. Dallas: American Heart Association; 1991.
17. Mann G, Hankey GJ, Cameron D. Swallowing function after stroke: prognosis and prognostic factors at 6 months. Stroke 1999;30:744–8.

18. Smithard DG, O'Neill PA, Parks C, et al. Complications and outcome after acute stroke. Does dysphagia matter? Stroke 1996;27:1200–4.

19. Crary MA, Groher ME. Reinstituting oral feeding in tube-fed adult patients with dysphagia. Nutr Clin Pract 2006;21:576–86.

20. Manly JJ, Jones RN, Langa KM, et al. Estimating the prevalence of dementia and mild cognitive impairment in the US: the 2016 health and retirement study harmonized cognitive assessment protocol project. JAMA Neurol 2022;79(12):1242–9.

21. Groher ME, Crary MA. Dysphagia: clinical management in adults and children. Maryland Heights, MO: Mosby Elsevier; 2010.

22. Marik PE, Kaplan D. Aspiration pneumonia and dysphagia in the elderly. Chest 2003;124:328–36.

23. Ertekin C, Aydogdu I, Yuceyar N, et al. Pathophysiological mechanisms of oropharyngeal dysphagia in amyotrophic lateral sclerosis. Brain 2000;123:125–40.

24. Mayhew AJ, Amog K, Phillips S, et al. The prevalence of sarcopenia in community-dwelling older adults, an exploration of differences between studies and within definitions: A systematic review and meta-analyses. Age Ageing 2019;48:48–56.

25. Grant MD, Rudberg MA, Brody JA. Gastrostomy placement and mortality among hospitalized Medicare beneficiaries. JAMA 1998;279:1973–6, 88.

26. Roche V. Percutaneous endoscopic gastrostomy. Clinical care of PEG tubes in older adults. Geriatrics 2003;58(22–26):28–9, 89.

27. Robbins J, Gangnon RE, Theis SM, et al. The effects of lingual exercise on swallowing in older adults. J Am Geriatr Soc 2005;53:1483–9.

28. Chen YC, Chen PY, Wang YC, et al. Decreased swallowing function in the sarcopenic elderly without clinical dysphagia: a cross-sectional study. BMC Geriatr 2020;20:419.

29. Kuroda Y, Kuroda R. Relationship between thinness and swallowing function in Japanese older adults: implications for sarcopenic dysphagia. J Am Geriatr Soc 2012;60:1785–6.

30. Bryant M. Biofeedback in the treatment of a selected dysphagic patient. Dysphagia 1991;6:140–4.

31. Steele CM. Optimal approaches for measuring tongue-pressure functional reserve. J Aging Res 2013;2013:542909.

32. Caruso C, Candore G, Cigna D, et al. Cytokine production pathway in the elderly. Immunol Res 1996;15:84–90.

33. Marcott S, Dewan K, Kwan M, et al. Where dysphagia begins: polypharmacy and xerostomia. Fed Pract 2020 May;37(5):234–41.

34. Qato DM, Wilder J, Schumm LP, et al. Changes in prescription and over-the-counter medication and dietary supplement use among older adults in the United States, 2005 vs 2011. JAMA Intern Med 2016;176(4):473–82.

35. Vergis EN, Brennen C, Wagener M, et al. Pneumonia in long-term care: a prospective case-control study of risk factors and impact on survival. Arch Intern Med 2001;161:2378–81.

36. Bivona PL. Xerostomia. A common problem among the elderly. N Y State Dent J 1998;64(6):46–52.

37. Ladenheim SE, Marlowe FI. Dysphagia secondary to cervical osteophytes. Am J Otolaryngol 1999;20:184–9.

38. Ekberg O, Hamdy S, Woisard V, et al. Social and psychological burden of dysphagia: its impact on diagnosis and treatment. Dysphagia 2002;17:139–46.

39. Wirth R, Dziewas R, Beck AM, et al. Oropharyngeal dysphagia in older persons—from pathophysiology to adequate intervention: A review and summary of an international expert meeting. Clin Interv Aging 2016;11:189–208.
40. Cereda E, Pedrolli C, Klersy C, et al. Nutritional status in older persons according to healthcare setting: A systematic review and meta-analysis of prevalence data using MNA(®). Clin. Nutr 2016;35:1282–90.
41. Pontoppidan H, Beecher HK. Progressive loss of protective reflexes in the airway with the advance in age. JAMA 1960;174:2209–13.
42. Michielsen W, Vandevondele D, Verschraegen G, et al. Bacterial surveillance cultures in a geriatric ward. Age Ageing 1993;22:221–6.
43. Sveinbjornsdottir S, Gudmundsson S, Briem H. Oropharyngeal colonization in the elderly. Eur J Clin Microbiol Infect Dis 1991;10:959–63.
44. Terpenning M, Bretz W, Lopatin D, et al. Bacterial colonization of saliva and plaque in the elderly. Clin Infect Dis 1993;16:S314–6.
45. Smithard DG, O'Neill PA, England RE, et al. The natural history of dysphagia following a stroke. Dysphagia 1997;12:188–93.
46. Masiero S, Pierobon R, Previato C, et al. Pneumonia in stroke patients with oropharyngeal dysphagia: a six-month follow-up study. Neurol Sci 2008;29:139–45.
47. Hoy M, Domer A, Plowman EK, et al. Causes of dysphagia in a tertiary-care swallowing center. Ann Otol Rhinol Laryngol 2013;122:335–8.
48. Kuhn M, Belafsky P. Management of cricopharyngeus muscle dysfunction. Otolaryngol Clin N Am 2013;46:1087–99.
49. Randall DR, Evangelista LM, Kuhn MA, et al. Improved symptomatic, functional, and fluoroscopic outcomes following serial "series of three" double-balloon dilation for cricopharyngeus muscle dysfunction. J Otolaryngol Head Neck Surg 2018;47(1):35.
50. Park RH, Allison MC, Lang J, et al. Randomized comparison of percutaneous endoscopic gastrostomy and nasogastric tube feeding in patients with persisting neurological dysphagia. BMJ 1992;304:1406–9.

Zebras in Adult Dysphagia Workup

Where to Look When You Think You Have Looked Everywhere

Melin Tan-Geller, MD*

KEYWORDS

- Globus • Cricopharyngeal spasm • No burp syndrome • Muscle tension dysphagia
- Xerostomia • Functional dysphagia

KEY POINTS

- Not all patients who have significant quality of life compromise from dysphagia have identifiable pathology in objective testing.
- For patients whose dysphagia etiology is unclear, keen clinical evaluation is of utmost importance.
- Despite seemingly normal exam findings and normal objective testing, consideration for disorders of the upper esophageal sphincter should be considered.
- A holistic approach with consideration for additional therapies may relieve functional and psychogenic dysphagia.

INTRODUCTION

Swallowing is a seemingly simple yet deceptively complex process of neuromuscular complexity, all of which can lead to nonspecific symptoms that are broad in range. While many pathologic processes that cause dysphagia have a distinct constellation of symptoms, often a patient presents with symptoms of dysphagia without apparent pathology. It is not uncommon to have a patient who has consistent and persistent discomfort with swallowing, who has been seen by several clinicians with unconcerning examination findings and whose objective testing yields no significant pathology. Despite the large range of pathology that can affect swallowing, much of swallowing occurs deeper than the surface of what we see in examination. In an evaluation of subjective dysphagia as it correlates to objective testing, 20% of 75 patients in the cohort had abnormal laryngeal examination findings, suggesting that another 80%

Department of Otorhinolaryngology–Head and Neck Surgery, Albert Einstein College of Medicine/Montefiore Medical Center, Bronx, NY, USA
* ENT & Allergy Associates, 222 Bloomingdale Road Suite 205, White Plains, NY 10605.
E-mail address: mtangeller@entandallergy.com

Otolaryngol Clin N Am 57 (2024) 695–701
https://doi.org/10.1016/j.otc.2024.03.001
0030-6665/24/© 2024 Elsevier Inc. All rights reserved.

had normal laryngoscopic examination findings.[1] However, in this study, there was a significant correlation between subjective quality of life dysphagia scores when compared to objective testing including videofluoroscopic swallow studies and flexible endoscopic evaluations of swallow. While most pathologic causes of dysphagia can be clarified with objective studies, not all patients who have significant quality of life compromise from dysphagia have identifiable pathology, leaving us with a diagnostic conundrum. The aim of this article is to review possible etiologies of dysphagia when objective evidence of dysphagia is lacking. Included in this discussion is cricopharyngeal spasm, retrograde cricopharyngeal dysfunction (R-CPD), muscle tension dysphagia, the effect of medications on swallowing, and functional dysphagia.

DISCUSSION
Globus

Any discussion of dysphagia with an elusive diagnosis requires the mention of globus pharyngeus. Globus is the sensation of having a lump in the throat. Up to 45% of the general population will report a mild or intermittent globus sensation at some point in their lives, and it accounts for up to 4% of new otolaryngology outpatient visits.[2] While the etiology of globus has been exhaustively studied, it is still poorly understood. Among many propositions, globus has been most attributed to reflux.[3-5] It also seems that for every study that claims a cause such as reflux, there is another study that refutes it.[6-8] However, patients who present with globus pharyngeus often have a subjective dysphagia with no clear etiology. Diagnostic criteria for globus must include the following: (1) Persistent or intermittent, nonpainful sensation of a lump or foreign body in the throat with no structural lesion identified on physical examination, laryngoscopy, or endoscopy; (2) Occurrence of the sensation between meals; (3) Absence of dysphagia or odynophagia; (4) Absence of a gastric inlet patch in the proximal esophagus; (5) Absence of evidence that gastroesophageal reflux or eosinophilic esophagitis is the cause of the symptom; and (6) Absence of major esophageal motor disorders.[9] Essentially, globus is a prominent symptom in the absence of any clear unequivocal diagnosis.

Cricopharyngeal Dysfunction

One commonly accepted explanation for the symptom of globus is cricopharyngeal dysfunction. The upper esophageal sphincter (UES) is composed of the most inferior fibers of the inferior constrictor muscle, the horizontal and oblique fibers of the cricopharyngeus (CP) muscle, and the most superior part of the cervical esophagus. The horizontal fibers of the CP encircle the upper esophagus, and at rest, they are tonically contracted. The idea that globus may represent a spasm of the CP muscle was first demonstrated by Watson in 1974 who showed that 9 patients with globus had elevated UES pressures compared to 22 control subjects.[10] Subsequent studies have supported this.[7,8] Dysphagia attributed to CP muscle dysfunction represents a range of severity on a continuum from CP hypertonicity to Zenker's diverticulum and is typically apparent in radiographs and manometry. Elevated sphincteric pressures are detected in manometry due to increased UES resting pressure, incomplete UES relaxation, incomplete UES opening, and incoordination of pharyngeal contractions and UES opening.[11] However, CP dysfunction may be spastic, intermittent, and therefore not always apparent. The diagnosis of CP spasm requires a high index of suspicion despite lack of pathology seen in testing. Not only is CP spasm a diagnostic challenge but also treatment is a challenge. Moving forward with treatment of a diagnosis based on suspicion is a leap of faith. Botox injection of the CP muscle, dilation, or myotomy are the methods of treatment of cricopharyngeal dysfunction.

Dilation is the least studied of the 3 treatments although it is favored as a first surgical step prior to the more morbid myotomy, and it is seen to be effective.[12,13] Cricopharyngeal myotomy is the gold standard treatment, and its success rate is seen to be significantly higher than that of botox injection but not significantly higher than that of dilation.[14] However, botox injection is a safer option, albeit temporary, and helpful where the dysphagia diagnosis is elusive.[15] Due to the minimal invasiveness of the procedure, decreased morbidity, and the ability to perform it in the clinic setting using electromyography (EMG) guidance, many advocate for botox injection over myotomy.[16] A range of 5 to 100 units have been reported to be successful.[15,17–19]

Retrograde Cricopharyngeal Dysfunction/"No Burp" Syndrome

In contrast to cricopharyngeal dysfunction, the diagnosis of R-CPD was borne out of a case series published by Bastian and colleagues in which a common symptom among patient with otherwise diffuse digestive symptoms was the inability to burp.[20] Patients experienced a wide range of swallowing complaints with the common denominator being the inability to burp, giving rise to the name no burp syndrome. With compromised CP muscle relaxation, retrograde gas release is compromised and patients also experience uncontrolled gurgling noises from the throat along with discomfort along the path of the esophagus and abdomen. Also common among patients in the Bastian cohort was an extensive prior otolaryngologic and gastroenterologic evaluation yielding normal examination findings and normal test results. The same group later described a case series of 200 patients seeking treatment of dysphagia, 81.1% of whom had already undergone at least 1 diagnostic procedure or therapy and 53.5% of which had been given empiric trials of medications. Additionally, the majority had also undergone gastrointestinal endoscopy. Any prior testing had been deemed "normal," and if treatment was provided, it did not resolve symptoms. One could sum that patients with R-CPD not only universally experienced inability to burp but also that the prior evaluations, diagnostic testing, and therapy yielded no clear prior diagnosis.[21] Each patient had been a diagnostic conundrum until the diagnosis of R-CPD was made. R-CPD diagnosis is made exclusively by syndromic presentation. Treatment is cricopharyngeal botox injection. In the operating room setting, performed endoscopically, injection of 30 to 80 units of botox is successful in providing initial relief of symptoms is 88% to 95% of the patient population based on 3 published reports thus far.[22–24] Alternatively, CP botox injection in the office setting is safe and does not require general anesthesia. However, the success rate in the office setting using 30 units of botox is 64.9% of 37 patients based on one institution's experience.[24] Alternatively, partial CP myotomy with a division of approximately 80% of the CP muscle has been proposed in a case report for those whose symptoms resolve with botox injection but whose resolution is limited.[22] In theory, complete CP myotomy would likely yield excellent symptomatic relief; however, in this case report, a portion of the muscle was left intact in order to avoid perforation and complication. As the recognition of R-CPD becomes more widely spread and understood, more investigation regarding the dosing of botox and alternative intervention is likely to hone the management of this patient population.

Muscle Tension Dysphagia

Another nascent dysphagia concept is muscle tension dysphagia (MTDg). Kang and colleagues introduced MTDg in 2016 in a case series of patients who experienced idiopathic dysphagia with normal videofluoroscopic swallow studies but with evident muscle tension seen in laryngoscopy.[25] In a subsequent study, the authors further defined the patient population to have normal esophagogastroduodenoscopy, high-resolution esophageal manometry with stationary impedance, and Bravo pH Probe off proton pump inhibitors.[26] The most prominent patient symptoms include globus (33% of 20 patients), difficulty swallowing solids, throat discomfort when swallowing, and sensation of food sticking in the throat, all of which are nonspecific and can be multifactorial. Additional symptoms include coughing or choking while eating and aberrant sounds when eating. Eighty-two percent of 20 patients exhibited signs or symptoms of laryngeal hyperresponsiveness. While there is an association between laryngeal muscle tension and the dysphagic symptoms, the examination findings of laryngeal muscle tension are subjective and clinician dependent. An astute clinician with an index of suspicion for muscle tension is needed to arrive at a diagnosis of MTDg. Patients may be treated effectively with speech language pathology intervention. Alternatively, laryngeal manipulation may also be of benefit.[27]

Xerostomia

Any disease state or medication that causes xerostomia may adversely affect swallow. Salivary gland hypoplasia can be objectively determined by sialometry, demonstrating decreased saliva production. However, in the absence of this, dry mouth is difficult to quantify. Moreover, there are no studies to correlate the degree of xerostomia with dysphagia. Dry mouth, however, contributes to dysphagia purely by decreasing lubrication to the oral and pharyngeal mucosa required to masticate and initiate the first stages of deglutition. Whether dysphagia can be attributed to diminished saliva and oropharyngeal dryness alone has yet to be elucidated.

However, Belafsky and Postma proposed a cycle of reflux in patients with Sjogren's syndrome that starts with xerostomia.[28] The limited buffering from saliva makes the esophagus more vulnerable to the deleterious effects of prolonged acid contact, which may in turn impair esophageal motility and reduce acid clearance.

By extension, any cause of xerostomia may lead to dysphagia in the same way. Pharmacology is a leading cause of dry mouth sensation as several classes of both prescription and nonprescription medications that have this undesirable effect. Anticholinergic, antihistamine, antidepressant, neuroleptic, antihypertensive, antiparkinsonian, antidiarrheal, and antiemetic medications have anticholinergic side effects that cause secondary decreased production of saliva. Alcohol effectively acts as a diuretic and may be factored into the dysphagia equation as well. Alternatively, cholinergic antagonists, cholinesterases, and benzodiazepines can also challenge normal swallowing with hypersalivation. Salivary flow can also be affected in patients with high levels of anxiety and related increased sympathetic nervous system activation.[29]

Broader consideration of pharmacology is warranted in patients with an elusive etiology of dysphagia. Beyond medications that contribute to xerostomia, medications that affect mental status such as sedatives, neuroleptic, and anticonvulsant medications may alter the swallowing mechanism by altering overall muscular tone and coordination.[30] Additionally, common medications such as calcium channel blockers, benzodiazepines, and theophylline may diminish lower esophageal sphincter tone and promote gastroesophageal reflux disease. Polypharmacy is not uncommon among the elderly.[30,31] Medications are more slowly metabolized in elderly, and therefore, pharmaceuticals can potentiate further swallow challenges in the aged population.[30] Making patients aware of the effects of medication in combination of any other contributing pathology may allow for counteractive measures against the undesirable side effects that affect the swallowing mechanism.

Phagophobia and Psychogenic Dysphagia

Phagophobia or fear of swallowing, like all phobias, is an anxiety disorder. Also known as choking phobia or swallowing phobia, it is characterized by a sensation of inability to swallow without the presence of any physical abnormality.[32] In one study juxtaposing eating disorders with phagophobia, those with psychogenic dysphagia did not appear to have an eating disorder; however, they did have clinically significant psychological distress.[33] In these cases, psychological evaluation with psychotherapy is the mainstay of treatment.

Functional Dysphagia

Functional dysphagia is a sensation of abnormal bolus transit through the esophageal body in the absence of structural, mucosal, or motility disorders to explain symptoms.[34] Functional dysphagia is distinctly exclusive of motility or structural disease and is a diagnosis of exclusion after exhaustive investigation including endoscopy and proton-pump inhibitor trials. Because it is a diagnosis of exclusion, an algorithmic approach to this diagnosis has been recommended.[35] Visceral hypersensitivity is thought to be a potential cause of functional gastrointestinal disorders. Varying studies indicate that mechanical stimuli in the gut may be inappropriately interpreted as painful due to a disturbance in the brain–gut axis.[35] Antidepressant medications may provide visceral anesthesia.[36] Brain–gut behavioral therapy, which includes hypnotherapy and cognitive behavioral therapy, may be of benefit to this patient population.[37] Ultimately, the treatment of functional dysphagia rests with reassurance and emphasis on the benign nature of the disease.

SUMMARY

While many patients who present with dysphagia have a clinically identifiable cause of dysphagia, the etiology of swallowing difficulty is oftentimes a diagnostic enigma. Functional dysphagia is diagnosed when no apparent pathology is identified and is based on clearly delineated criteria. When the symptoms of dysphagia are disproportionate to the objective findings, consideration for muscular dysfunction as seen in disorders of the CP muscle and MTDg should rise high in the differential diagnosis. Additionally, pharmacologic effects of varying medications may play a role as well. When the etiology of dysphagia remains a mystery, the diagnosis relies heavily on patient history. It behooves us to remain astute history-takers and to maintain a wide lens of observations in our physical examinations when evaluating patients with dysphagia.

CLINICS CARE POINTS

- CP spasm may be intermittent and inconsistent and therefore clinically evasive.
- The diagnosis of R-CPD, also known as no burp syndrome, is made by patient history alone, and therefore, a high index of suspicion is warranted.
- Globus may represent CP muscle dysfunction or MTDg, both of which also require a high index of suspicion.
- Any disease state or medication that causes xerostomia may contribute to dysphagia.
- Myriad classes of prescription and nonprescription medications can adversely affect swallowing.
- Functional dysphagia is distinctly exclusive of motility or structural disease and is a diagnosis of exclusion after exhaustive investigation including endoscopy and proton-pump inhibitor trials.

DISCLOSURE

The author has nothing to disclose.

REFERENCES

1. Dewan K, Clarke JO, Kamal AN, et al. Patient reported outcomes and objective swallowing assessments in a multidisciplinary dysphagia clinic. Laryngoscope 2021;131(5):1088–94.
2. Moloy PJ, Charter R. The globus symptom. Incidence, therapeutic response, and age and sex relationships. Arch Otolaryngol 1982;108(11):740–4.
3. Hill J, Stuart RC, Fung HK, et al. Gastroesophageal reflux, motility disorders, and psychological profiles in the etiology of globus pharyngis. Laryngoscope 1997; 107(10):1373–7.
4. Koufman JA. The otolaryngologic manifestations of gastroesophageal reflux disease (GERD): a clinical investigation of 225 patients using ambulatory 24-hour pH monitoring and an experimental investigation of the role of acid and pepsin in the development of laryngeal injury. Laryngoscope 1991;101(4 Pt 2 Suppl 53):1–78.
5. Smit CF, et al. Gastropharyngeal and gastroesophageal reflux in globus and hoarseness. Arch Otolaryngol Head Neck Surg 2000;126(7):827–30.
6. Chen CL, Tsai CC, Chou ASB, et al. Utility of ambulatory pH monitoring and videofluoroscopy for the evaluation of patients with globus pharyngeus. Dysphagia 2007;22(1):16–9.
7. Corso MJ, Pursnani KG, Mohiuddin MA, et al. Globus sensation is associated with hypertensive upper esophageal sphincter but not with gastroesophageal reflux. Dig Dis Sci 1998;43(7):1513–7.
8. Wilson JA, Heading RC, Maran AG, et al. Globus sensation is not due to gastrooesophageal reflux. Clin Otolaryngol Allied Sci 1987;12(4):271–5.
9. Drossman DA, Hasler WL. Rome IV-Functional GI Disorders: Disorders of Gut-Brain Interaction. Gastroenterology 2016;150(6):1257–61.
10. Watson WC, Sullivan SN. Hypertonicity of the cricopharyngeal sphincter: A cause of globus sensation. Lancet 1974;2(7894):1417–9.
11. Veenker EA, Andersen PE, Cohen JI. Cricopharyngeal spasm and Zenker's diverticulum. Head Neck 2003;25(8):681–94.
12. Clary MS, Daniero JJ, Keith SW, et al. Efficacy of large-diameter dilatation in cricopharyngeal dysfunction. Laryngoscope 2011;121(12):2521–5.
13. Solt J, Bajor J, Moizs M, et al. Primary cricopharyngeal dysfunction: treatment with balloon catheter dilatation. Gastrointest Endosc 2001;54(6):767–71.
14. Kocdor P, Siegel ER, Tulunay-Ugur OE. Cricopharyngeal dysfunction: A systematic review comparing outcomes of dilatation, botulinum toxin injection, and myotomy. Laryngoscope 2016;126(1):135–41.
15. Blitzer A, Brin MF. Use of botulinum toxin for diagnosis and management of cricopharyngeal achalasia. Otolaryngol Head Neck Surg 1997;116(3):328–30.
16. Schneider I, Thumfart WF, Pototschnig C, et al. Treatment of dysfunction of the cricopharyngeal muscle with botulinum A toxin: introduction of a new, noninvasive method. Ann Otol Rhinol Laryngol 1994;103(1):31–5.
17. Alberty J, Oelerich M, Ludwig K, et al. Efficacy of botulinum toxin A for treatment of upper esophageal sphincter dysfunction. Laryngoscope 2000;110(7):1151–6.
18. Haapaniemi JJ, Laurikainen EA, Pulkkinen J, et al. Botulinum toxin in the treatment of cricopharyngeal dysphagia. Dysphagia 2001;16(3):171–5.

19. Terre R, Valles M, Panades A, et al. Long-lasting effect of a single botulinum toxin injection in the treatment of oropharyngeal dysphagia secondary to upper esophageal sphincter dysfunction: a pilot study. Scand J Gastroenterol 2008;43(11): 1296–303.

20. Bastian RW, Smithson ML. Inability to Belch and Associated Symptoms Due to Retrograde Cricopharyngeus Dysfunction: Diagnosis and Treatment. OTO Open 2019;3(1). 2473974X19834553.

21. Hoesli RC, Wingo ML, Bastian RW. The Long-term Efficacy of Botulinum Toxin Injection to Treat Retrograde Cricopharyngeus Dysfunction. OTO Open 2020;4(2). 2473974X20938342.

22. Bastian RW, Hoesli RC. Partial Cricopharyngeal Myotomy for Treatment of Retrograde Cricopharyngeal Dysfunction. OTO Open 2020;4(2). 2473974X20917644.

23. Siddiqui SH, Sagalow ES, Fiorella MA, et al. Retrograde Cricopharyngeus Dysfunction: The Jefferson Experience. Laryngoscope 2023;133(5):1081–5.

24. Doruk C, Pitman MJ. Lateral transcervical in-office botulinum toxin injection for retrograde cricopharyngeal dysfunction. Laryngoscope 2024;134(1):283–6.

25. Kang CH, Hentz JG, Lott DG. Muscle tension dysphagia: symptomology and theoretical framework. Otolaryngol Head Neck Surg 2016;155(5):837–42.

26. Kang CH, Zhang N, Lott DG. Muscle tension dysphagia: contributing factors and treatment efficacy. Ann Otol Rhinol Laryngol 2021;130(7):674–81.

27. DePietro JD, Rubin S, Stein DJ, et al. Laryngeal manipulation for dysphagia with muscle tension dysphonia. Dysphagia 2018;33(4):468–73.

28. Belafsky PC, Postma GN. The laryngeal and esophageal manifestations of Sjogren's syndrome. Curr Rheumatol Rep 2003;5(4):297–303.

29. Broniatowski M, Sonies BC, Rubin JS, et al. Current evaluation and treatment of patients with swallowing disorders. Otolaryngol Head Neck Surg 1999;120(4): 464–73.

30. Schindler JS, Kelly JH. Swallowing disorders in the elderly. Laryngoscope 2002; 112(4):589–602.

31. Marcott S, Dewan K, Kwan M, et al. Where Dysphagia Begins: Polypharmacy and Xerostomia. Fed Pract 2020;37(5):234–41.

32. Baijens LW, Koetsenruijter K, Pilz W. Diagnosis and treatment of phagophobia: a review. Dysphagia 2013;28(2):260–70.

33. Barofsky I, Fontaine KR. Do psychogenic dysphagia patients have an eating disorder? Dysphagia 1998;13(1):24–7.

34. Drossman DA. Functional gastrointestinal disorders: history, pathophysiology, clinical features and Rome IV. Gastroenterology 2016. https://doi.org/10.1053/j.gastro.2016.02.032.

35. Baumann A, Katz PO. Functional disorders of swallowing. Handb Clin Neurol 2016;139:483–8.

36. Weijenborg PW, de Schepper HS, Smout AJPM, et al. Effects of antidepressants in patients with functional esophageal disorders or gastroesophageal reflux disease: a systematic review. Clin Gastroenterol Hepatol 2015;13(2):251–259 e1.

37. Luo Y, Keefer L. The Clinical value of brain-gut behavioral therapies for functional esophageal disorders and symptoms. Neuro Gastroenterol Motil 2022;34(6): e14373.

Printed and bound by CPI Group (UK) Ltd, Croydon, CR0 4YY

03/10/2024

01040476-0017